T0210731

DIAGNOSTIC CULTURES

Classical and Contemporary Social Theory

Series Editor: Stjepan G. Mestrovic, Texas A&M University, USA

Classical and Contemporary Social Theory publishes rigorous scholarly work that re-discovers the relevance of social theory for contemporary times, demonstrating the enduring importance of theory for modern social issues. The series covers social theory in a broad sense, inviting contributions on both 'classical' and modern theory, thus encompassing sociology, without being confined to a single discipline. As such, work from across the social sciences is welcome, provided that volumes address the social context of particular issues, subjects, or figures and offer new understandings of social reality and the contribution of a theorist or school to our understanding of it. The series considers significant new appraisals of established thinkers or schools, comparative works or contributions that discuss a particular social issue or phenomenon in relation to the work of specific theorists or theoretical approaches. Contributions are welcome that assess broad strands of thought within certain schools or across the work of a number of thinkers, but always with an eye toward contributing to contemporary understandings of social issues and contexts.

Also in the series

A Sociology of the Total Organization
Atomistic Unity in the French Foreign Legion
Mikaela Sundberg
ISBN 978-1-4724-5560-4

Arendt Contra Sociology
Theory, Society and its Science
Philip Walsh
ISBN 978-1-4094-3863-2

Being Human in a Consumer Society
Edited by Alejandro Néstor García Martínez
ISBN 978-1-4724-4317-5

Diagnostic Cultures
A Cultural Approach to the Pathologization
of Modern Life

SVEND BRINKMANN
Aalborg University, Denmark

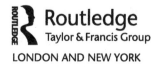

Routledge
Taylor & Francis Group

LONDON AND NEW YORK

First published 2016 by Routledge

2 Park Square, Milton Park, Abingdon, Oxfordshire OX14 4RN
52 Vanderbilt Avenue, New York, NY 10017

Routledge is an imprint of the Taylor & Francis Group, an informa business

First issued in paperback 2020

British Library Cataloguing in Publication Data
A catalogue record for this book is available from the British Library

Library of Congress Cataloging in Publication Data
Brinkmann, Svend
    Diagnostic cultures : a cultural approach to the pathologization of modern life / by Svend Brinkmann.
        pages cm. — (Classical and contemporary social theory)
    Includes bibliographical references and index.
        ISBN 978-1-4724-1319-2 (hardback) — ISBN 978-1-4724-1320-8 (ebook) — ISBN 978-1-4724-1321-5 (epub)   1. Mental illness—Diagnosis.   2. Social psychiatry.   3. Social psychology.   I. Title.
    RC469.B75 2016
    616.89'071—dc23
    2015033034

ISBN: 978-1-4724-1319-2 (hbk)
ISBN: 978-0-367-59688-0 (pbk)

Typeset in Times New Roman
by Apex CoVantage, LLC

Contents

List of Figures

Acknowledgements

I wish to thank Anders Petersen, Ester Holte Kofod, Mikka Nielsen, Mette Rønberg, Andreas Kjær, Rolf Lyneborg Lund and Rasmus Birk, who have been close collaborators in different ways on the research project Diagnostic Culture, which forms the background to the analyses of the present book. I have presented and discussed most of the ideas of the book with these excellent researchers, and I am grateful for their comments and criticisms. Some of them read the entire manuscript and provided very valuable feedback. I would also like to thank Jaan Valsiner for his thoughts on cultural psychology and for being open to my ideas of how to develop this line of thought into a theory about mental disorder. I am extremely grateful that the Danish Council for Independent Research decided to fund our work on diagnostic cultures (Grant no. 12-125597), which enabled me not only to do much more empirical and theoretical research than I could otherwise have done (and also employ excellent doctoral students), but which also made it possible for me to travel and spend time at King's College London (thanks to Nikolas Rose for welcoming me there). Furthermore I want to thank Neil Jordan from Ashgate for taking an interest in my ideas very early on and for encouraging me to develop them into a book manuscript. I also owe a big thank you to numerous reviewers and editors of articles and book chapters that I have written in the course of preparing the current manuscript, and many of the chapters are based on (or recycle some) materials that have been published in different versions before:

Brinkmann, S. (in press). Towards a cultural psychology of mental disorder: The case of ADHD. *Culture & Psychology*.

Brinkmann, S. (2014). Languages of suffering. *Theory & Psychology*, 24(5), 630–648.

Brinkmann, S. (2014). Psychiatric diagnoses as semiotic mediators: The case of ADHD. *Nordic Psychology*, 66(2), 121–134.

Brinkmann, S. (2013). The pathologization of morality. In K. Keohane & A. Petersen (Eds) *The Social Pathologies of Contemporary Civilization*. Farnham: Ashgate.

Brinkmann, S. (2012). The mind as skills and dispositions: On normativity and mediation. *Integrative Psychological and Behavioral Science*, 46(1), 78–89.

Brinkmann, S. (2011). Towards an expansive hybrid psychology: Integrating theories of the mediated mind. *Integrative Psychological and Behavioral Science*, 45(1), 1–20.

Brinkmann, S. (2005). Human kinds and looping effects in psychology: Foucauldian and hermeneutic perspectives. *Theory & Psychology*, 15(6), 769–791.

Introduction

Psychiatric diagnoses such as depression, anxiety, autism and ADHD have today become ever-present in our conversations about our problems: they operate as powerful categories in the social and health systems of modern welfare states, and they have entered public media and popular culture. The concepts of illness and disorder – and the diagnoses with which we designate our problems – are no longer just medical, biological and psychological concepts, but also bureaucratic, social and administrative entities (Rosenberg, 2007, p. 5). McGann goes so far as to conclude that "diagnoses have become part of how we make sense of ourselves, each other, and the world" (McGann, 2011, p. 343). The purpose of this book is to describe and analyse this phenomenon, which I refer to as the development of diagnostic cultures.

Huge amounts of money are involved in contemporary diagnostic cultures. The global cost of mental illness has been estimated at 2.5 trillion US dollars – a number that is expected to grow to a shocking 6 trillion dollars by 2030 (Kincaid & Sullivan, 2014, p. 1). Many studies estimate that around 25 per cent of the population in Western countries will suffer from at least one diagnosable mental disorder in the course of one year (Kessler, 2010). The estimated life time prevalence is usually set around 50 percent. According to many psychiatrists, this shows that their discipline has progressed to a stage where they are finally able to find, diagnose and treat the mentally ill that have always been there. Perhaps, for some disorders, there are more ill people than before, but overall, the argument goes, the difference between the old days and contemporary times is that we can now finally locate the ill and disordered. Some sociologists argue on the contrary that these numbers are proof that modern life creates new epidemics of social pathologies. Many more people are in fact mentally disordered than before, because we live in disordered times. The high numbers are a sign that something is deeply wrong in our culture. People in the West are rarely dying today because of material poverty, hunger or appalling physical working conditions – as in the times of Karl Marx – but they are suffering from various mental disorders, ranging from depression and anxiety to eating disorders and bipolar conditions, because of terrible and alienating circumstances of social life.

Without completely discarding these interpretations, I argue in this book that something more fundamental has been happening in recent years: the development of what I call diagnostic cultures. The concept of diagnostic cultures refers to the numerous ways that psychiatric categories are used by people – patients, professionals, and almost everyone else – to interpret, regulate and mediate various forms of self-understanding and activity. In the religious cultures of previous times, it was particularly religious concepts that mediated people's relationships to themselves and each other, and it was religious ideas that people mobilized to give meaning to their experienced suffering. Although religion has far from disappeared from our post-secular society (McLennan, 2010), it is now more often psychiatry and its diagnoses that are invoked to account for the problems that people experience. I thus follow in the footsteps of Bowker and Star, who, in their classic sociological account of how classifications work in society, pointed out that "classification has become a direct tool mediating human suffering" (Bowker & Star, 2000, p. 26). The concept of diagnostic cultures is meant to draw our attention to the many different ways that diagnoses mediate human suffering, and it is important to use the concept of cultures in the plural form, because this happens in quite different ways in different societal arenas.

In the present book, I intend to focus specifically on *psychiatric* diagnoses as classifications, and my goal is to analyse how diagnostic cultures become manifest in society at large, leading to a situation in which we increasingly interpret our sufferings in the light of psychiatric conceptions and diagnostic terminology. I say "we", because diagnostic cultures are not simply advocated by doctors and other professionals belonging to "the system". We can no longer, like the anti-psychiatric movement of the 1970s, simply accuse psychiatrists of promoting "medicalization from above" (saying that it is the doctors and "the system" that make us ill!), for patients and citizens themselves are increasingly pushing for "pathologization from below" (McGann, 2011), seeking diagnoses as explanations of various life problems. The point is that the recognition of the emergence of diagnostic cultures as a widespread and pervasive aspect of contemporary social life should lead us to discuss the opposition between the psychiatric (we can now finally locate the ill!) and the sociological (a disordered society makes us ill!) arguments in a different light. It is not that these arguments are faulty *per se* (indeed, both of them might contain more than a grain of truth), but they might concern superficial aspects of a more profound historical development and change in our very ideas of human distress.

This book aims to analyse and account for different aspects of contemporary diagnostic cultures. Based on a cultural psychological analysis – informed by sociology and cultural studies – and using ADHD in the adult population as the prime illustrative case study, it explains why there is, in an individualized and secularized age, a felt need to explain one's suffering, discomfort and problems in psychiatric terms. It also argues more critically that we risk losing vital resources of self-understanding if we continue to pathologize human suffering; that is, approach suffering largely in terms of illness or disorder. Existential, political and moral concerns are today easily transformed into individual psychiatric disorders, and we thereby risk losing sight of the larger historical and social forces that affect our lives. This has severe consequences for our abilities to act in order to help people with their problems. Our actions are increasingly informed by diagnoses, which risks individualizing and de-contextualizing the problems that people have.

In addition to describing, analyzing and criticizing the phenomenon of diagnostic cultures, the book also provides a philosophical analysis of suffering and psychiatric problems, disorders and illnesses, and advocates a broad and non-reductive approach that highlights the idea that suffering can be much more than a mental health problem. It should also be seen in political, moral and existential terms. We should avoid narrowing down our conception of suffering to that which can be framed as "symptoms" on a checklist. We should in many cases counter the current pathologization of human life, but this presupposes a sociological understanding of diagnostic cultures, and it also calls for alternative conceptualizations of suffering that transcend diagnostic understandings.

This book is not just a descriptive account of diagnostic cultures, but also has the ambition of contributing to current social theory by introducing the theoretical framework of cultural psychology (e.g., Valsiner, 2007; 2014). Cultural psychology, although referred to *as* psychology, is actually an interdisciplinary form of social science (like cognitive science or neuroscience) that theorizes human action, thinking and feeling as semiotically mediated in social practices. Cultural psychology, in the version articulated here, integrates in particular social psychology with history and social and cultural theory, and I believe that this kind of integration is needed in order to capture both the ways in which social processes affect how individuals suffer and think about mental illness, and also how such social processes are shaped by problems and discontents experienced by human beings. In order to understand the diagnostic cultures of contemporary society, and human suffering more broadly, we need to understand how personal and cultural life is woven together; that is, how human beings are at the same time individually social and socially individual (Valsiner, 2014, p. 53). The scientific project of cultural psychology is to analyze exactly this, and it distinguishes itself from related perspectives (such as structuration paradigms or symbolic interactionism, for example) by its view of *persons* as the irreducible units of social life (Harré, 1983). I will return to that, but shall here make explicit some of the central aims of this book:

1. To chart the emerging diagnostic cultures in contemporary society and ask: how do psychiatric diagnoses affect modern society and people living today?
2. To analyze the impact of diagnostic cultures on our understanding of and means of coping with various human problems: how are diagnoses put to use by individuals who are diagnosed (or increasingly understand themselves in the light of diagnostic categories)?
3. To articulate a cultural psychological perspective (integrating social psychology, sociology and cultural studies) that is applicable to "clinical" phenomena (such as ADHD): how do personal problems interact with broader societal trends, and how can this be studied?
4. To critically question the distinction between nature and culture, biology and the social sciences, which is increasingly incapable of helping us explain

the sufferings that people feel in their lives today: if most mental disorders that are diagnosed represent entanglements of biological, psychological and social issues as these play out in the lives of acting and suffering persons, then how should mental disorder be defined and addressed (theoretically and in practice)?

The contents of the individual chapters are described more fully in what follows:

Chapter 1 centres on the concept of diagnostic culture itself and takes the reader through the diagnostic cultures of contemporary Western societies. It demonstrates how psychiatric diagnoses are affecting many corners of the social world from education and work to private life. The point is that we are increasingly taught to understand our problems and sufferings through a diagnostic language. This chapter also develops a cultural psychological approach suited to analyzing diagnostic cultures. While psychiatric diagnoses have been much discussed in recent years, especially since the publication of DSM-5 in 2013 (see e.g. Cooper, 2014), little work has been done to study the impact of psychiatry and its diagnoses on individuals and society from cultural perspectives. In order to do so, we need an adequate understanding of persons as cultural beings, which cultural psychology is capable of providing. The chapter ends by outlining some of the most significant lines of criticism that have been developed against psychiatric ideas, which is provides some background for the ensuing analyses.

Building on three dimensions of diagnoses (referred to as the having, being, and doing dimensions), Chapter 2 provides an introduction to psychiatric diagnoses as epistemic objects; that is, objects of knowledge. Are genuine mental disorders pre-existing "objects" that one may *have* or not, in relative independence of diagnostic categories? Or could it be that disorders emerge in the world together with the diagnostic categories that point them out? Are we forced to choose between essentialism (the idea that diagnoses refer to pre-existing, disease-specific objects) and social constructionism (the idea that diagnoses construct diseases and disorders)? Or can we articulate a third possibility? How one answers these questions depends on one's conception of diagnoses as *epistemic objects*; that is, as objects of scientific knowledge and intervention. I introduce Ian Hacking's influential account of looping effects between categories and categorized, and present a sociological account of how a problem becomes taken up as a psychiatric disorder.

In Chapter 3, I argue that the diagnostic language (with its potentially pathologizing effects) is merely one among a large number of languages of suffering available to human beings when they try to make sense of their distress. The diagnostic language may have gained a certain hegemony in modern society, but religious, existential, moral and political languages are still around as part of our vocabulary, and in many ways needed in order to understand the different forms of human suffering and discomfort. This chapter therefore seeks to go against the diagnostic narrowing of our self-understanding by locating other discursive resources for understanding suffering.

In cultural psychology, semiotic mediation refers to persons' use of signs to regulate thoughts, acts and emotions. Based on fieldwork among adults diagnosed with ADHD, the fourth chapter highlights three specific functions that psychiatric diagnoses have today as semiotic mediators in the lives of the diagnosed: (1) An *explanatory* function in relation to experienced problems (even if a diagnosis is a description of symptoms, it is often used to explain these very symptoms), (2) a *self-affirming* function (in the sense that a diagnosis provides a framework according to which numerous phenomena appear as "symptoms"), and (3) a *disclaiming* function in relation to responsibility (with the possibility of medicalizing certain aspects of moral life). The legitimacy of each is discussed, which in itself might add to the distress experienced by adults categorized by a contested diagnosis such as ADHD.

"Do more, feel better, live longer" is the slogan of GlaxoSmithKline, one of the leading pharmaceutical companies in the world. Building on the idea that advertising is "the poetry of capitalism" that affects almost every corner of cultural life, Chapter 5 seeks to describe the kind of subject that is imagined and presupposed as ideal in a diagnostic culture (and a slogan like this). Doing *more* (no matter what?), feeling *better* (no matter why?), and living *longer* (no matter how?) are all quantitative indicators, which go hand in hand with the diagnostic approach to human problems. The diagnosed self easily becomes a quantitative entity, emptied of qualitative significance, which, however, has otherwise been highlighted as central to human self-understanding by cultural psychologists (and especially by the philosopher Charles Taylor). It is argued that the rush toward a quantified personhood can be seen as an attempt to create a kind of solidity in an era that Zygmunt Bauman has otherwise addressed as liquid modernity.

Chapter 6 outlines and discusses some of the most influential interpretations of the current "epidemics" of mental disorder in our diagnostic cultures. Are more people ill because of modern society? Have they always been ill, but are we only now able to find them because of scientific advances? Are the disorders fabricated by *Big Pharma*? I argue that these interpretations may be legitimate in certain cases, but that two others are more significant: the cultural-historical "psychiatrization" of suffering on the one hand and changed diagnostic practices on the other. What is often criticized as unwarranted pathologization comes in many forms today (e.g. as self-pathologization, but also as stigmatization), and it is argued in this chapter that "the pathologization of everything" is a huge problem for a number of reasons: it skews the resources available for treatment, it might paradoxically lead to increased vulnerability of individuals, it routinely individualizes social problems (thereby leading to individualized solutions in the form of pills or therapy) and it risks narrowing our self-understanding.

In order to inform the discussion of the current expansion of psychiatric diagnoses, I argue that we need to understand better the nature of mental disorders and psychiatric pathologies. What are these? This is a notoriously difficult question, and Chapter 7 begins by giving an outline of existing definitions from leading scholars and disciplines (Boorse, Wakefield, neuroscience, phenomenology, nominalism), and then I argue that the concept of mental disorder or illness is not held together by necessary and sufficient conditions, but by what Wittgenstein called family resemblance. Following from this, the chapter moves on to articulate an approach to the idea of mental disorder from a cultural psychological perspective. It is argued that cultural psychology has the potential to develop a comprehensive understanding of mental disorder that combines awareness of the brain and body with sociocultural norms and practices without reducing mental disorder to either of these. In that sense, it may steer a course between essentialist models of psychopathology on the one hand, and radical social constructionist ones on the other, in particular by putting the *person* (and not the brain or mind) at the centre of the theory. ADHD in adults is again referred to as an illustrative example, but the theory presented here has more general ambitions.

The final chapter sums up and looks to the future: Are we approaching the end of pathologization, becoming unable to locate further areas of pathology in diagnostic cultures, or will the future (with increasing uses of brain scans and genetic tests) only expand the diagnostic cultures further – even diagnosing before the symptoms appear, on the basis of risk calculations and genetic vulnerabilities?

Chapter 1

Introducing the Concept of Diagnostic Cultures

This chapter has two main purposes: first, I shall introduce the very idea of diagnostic cultures, which will be analyzed throughout the book, and second, I shall articulate the theoretical approach that will be used to analyze the phenomenon of diagnostic cultures. This approach is cultural psychology.

Living in Diagnostic Cultures

In one way, it should be quite easy to pinpoint the phenomenon of diagnostic cultures, because we (and when talking about "we", I include everyone in the imagined hemisphere we call the West, but also elsewhere on the planet) live in and with these cultures in almost every arena of social life, whenever people experience problems or act in ways that are considered deviant. Formal psychiatric diagnoses are not as old as one might think. The first edition of the diagnostic manual published by the American Psychiatric Association, called the DSM,[1] appeared as late as 1952, and although diagnostic terms were of course used before this time, it was only from the second half of the 20th century that psychiatric diagnoses really spread from practices in clinics and hospitals to schools, welfare organizations, and families. Today, most of us can use diagnostic terms such as depression, anxiety, bipolar, ADHD, PTSD and OCD, and also semi-diagnoses such as stress, when we talk about the problems that we or our children face in everyday life. We read self-help books about how to manage various psychological afflictions that can perhaps be diagnosed, and consume novels and television series (e.g. *The Sopranos*) in which the heroes or villains suffer from diagnosable mental disorders. When we open our newspapers, we are routinely confronted with frightening statistics that tell us, for example, that the WHO expects that depression will become the second leading cause of global disability by 2020; we learn that up to one quarter of the population is mentally ill within any one year; and we witness how pharmaceuticals against symptoms of depression, anxiety and ADHD are prescribed to more and more people – children and adults alike. Even in Denmark – allegedly the happiest nation in the world – more than eight per cent of the population consumes antidepressants, and for some age cohorts (especially older people), the number is dramatically higher.

---

1   The Diagnostic and Statistical Manual of Mental Disorders.

In what I call diagnostic cultures, psychiatric diagnoses are used by health professionals and lay people for many different purposes. Psychiatric terminology has been democratized and has travelled from the clinics and medical textbooks into popular culture (witness the example in Box 1.1).

Box 1.1   Mad or Normal? Psychiatric diagnoses as entertainment

In 2012 the national Danish Broadcasting Company aired the documentary "Mad or Normal?"[2] The idea was to challenge people's biases about the mentally ill by showing that they are in most respects "just like you and me". The show was run in an entertaining way, somewhat like a quiz, and hosted by a famous Danish "TV doctor": three experts (one psychiatrist, one psychologist and one psychiatric nurse) were confronted with a group of ten people they had not met before, and five of these people had different psychiatric diagnoses (schizophrenia, eating disorder, OCD, social phobia and bipolar depression). Through the episodes, the experts were supposed to match the diagnoses with five of the participants. The viewers could also participate by voting on the internet, trying to guess which of the participants were mentally ill. In order to help the experts and also the viewers in this guessing game, the participants had to go through a number of trials that were supposed to provide clues as to who were ill and who were well. For example, they had to perform stand-up comedy in front of a live audience (the idea being that this would be difficult for someone with social phobia), and do a farm animal clean up task (possibly revealing the OCD sufferer). But in fact – and seemingly in line with the programme's intentions – the experts could *not* guess who were ill, or which diagnoses belonged with whom. And the viewers were also quite poor at the guessing game.

What does a show like this tell us about diagnostic cultures and our complex attitudes to mental illness today? Initially, it can be observed that a show like this would have been quite unthinkable (at least in Denmark) just a few years ago. Psychiatric diagnoses were not publicly visible and would not be the centre of attention in a popular entertainment show on television. Superficially at least, this indicates that psychiatric problems are no longer taboo to the same extent and that stigmatization due to diagnoses has decreased. Furthermore, and in rather more subtle ways, the show points to a number of paradoxes inherent in the logics of the diagnostic cultures of the 21st century. For example, one powerful discourse, which is also mobilized in the television show, claims that

---

2   The show was a Danish adaptation of the BBC programme *How mad are you?* (See Progler, 2009, for a brief description and analysis from a medical science perspective.) Information on the Danish version can be found at: http://www.dr.dk/sundhed/Sygdom/ Psykiatri/Psykiatri.htm.

psychiatric problems are illnesses "just like somatic illnesses", as it is often said. In principle, there are no differences between somatic and psychiatric problems, and the two ought to be equal in the health care systems of the welfare state.[3] At the same time, the underlying logic of the show seems to go against this discourse of "illness equality". This can be seen if one imagines a similar show with people suffering from somatic illnesses. Would such a show be aired, with the participants having to go through trials that would bring forth their symptoms? This is very unlikely. Think of people with osteoporosis being forced to play hockey, for example, or diabetes patients eating loads of sweets. For some reason, it did not lead to public outcry (in fact quite the opposite) that people with mental disorders engaged in activities that were meant to disclose their illnesses. This reveals the contradictory understandings of psychiatric problems that we have in our diagnostic cultures: on the one hand, they are "just like somatic illnesses", but, on the other, they are clearly implicitly thought of as something else.

Related to this point, it was noteworthy that the people with diagnoses in the programme were said to be "not ill" at the time when the show was made. For ethical reasons it seems reasonable, of course, to only enrol people who are not overly vulnerable, and as a form of protection against the tests in the show, but, given this, it is hardly surprising that the experts and viewers were unable to guess who were suffering from the various mental disorders. Also in the book, which accompanied the television show, we hear that Kirstine (diagnosed with OCD) "is now cured", and she refers to her remaining problems as "bad habits, which everybody has" (Kyhn, 2012, p. 46). Again, to compare with somatic illness: if someone had once suffered a fracture, or had once had a tumour, but had since been cured, then no one would ever expect that people (not even experts) could come up with accurate guesses regarding these matters. So, although the programme meant to transmit the message that "they" are "just like us", it paradoxically came to implicitly conclude that "once a psychiatric patient, always a psychiatric patient" – even if the symptoms have disappeared. The premise of the show was that it should be possible to guess the disorders even though the (former) patients were now symptom free, so, contrary to its surely good intentions, the show came to reinforce a discourse of chronicity concerning psychiatric problems. Again, we see the contradictory logics operating in diagnostic cultures: on the one hand, we define and identify mental disorders on the basis of symptoms (which is something I shall return to a number of times in this book), but, on the

---

3   Recently, in Denmark, a "diagnosis guarantee" has been established, which means that patients have the right to obtain a diagnosis within one month of contacting the medical system. At first this guarantee did not pertain to psychiatric diagnoses, but this has now been changed, so that all kinds of health problems are put on an equal footing.

other, we hold the belief that such disorders may somehow persist even in the absence of manifest symptoms.

A couple of years later, in 2014, the show was followed up with two new episodes called "Mad or Normal? At the Job Interview" and, instead of mental health experts, three business managers were confronted with disguised psychiatric patients in a group of job applicants, and asked whom among the participants they would be interested in offering a job. Interestingly, the managers were very positive toward many of the people with diagnoses, and the "winner" was in fact a psychiatric patient. This second series, now thematizing psychiatric diagnoses and work life, demonstrates yet another paradoxical aspect of our diagnostic cultures: On the one hand, it is surely very positive that people who are diagnosed are considered "one of us" (which was the name of the accompanying national campaign to raise awareness about psychiatric disorders) to the extent that experts and business leaders cannot recognize them in a group of people. This can be seen as a demonstration that "they" *are* indeed "like us". However, they are still "they", and paradoxically identified as excluded through the diagnostic label. On the other hand, the argument or demonstration of just-like-us-ness can quickly be turned on its head to become a demonstration that if they are "just like us", then why do they need special welfare benefits, pensions and other societally sanctioned advantages? The accompanying book asks the question directly: "If the three experts in the program are incapable of guessing who among the ten participants suffer from which disorders, then how on earth should the rest of us be capable of guessing it?" (Kyhn, 2012, p. 9). It might be a good thing in an ethical sense that viewers discover that psychiatric patients are nice people without dramatic problems, but the downside is that it might at the same time become difficult for patients to explain their sufferings and legitimize their need for help. This illustrates a broader dilemma concerning psychiatric diagnoses that will surface in various ways in this book: diagnoses may on the one hand be stigmatizing and pathologizing (and thus something one might wish to avoid), but, on the other hand, the labelling they provide can bring certain advantages in the diagnostic cultures of welfare states, which explains why some people actively seek to be diagnosed.

Box 1.1 is about psychiatric diagnoses as entertainment, or perhaps more accurately, "edutainment" aired on a respected public service television channel in Denmark, and it is meant to illustrate some of the ways in which diagnoses are conceived in contemporary society. From this little example, we have seen that a number of paradoxes are likely to emerge when dealing with psychiatric diagnoses today: (1) Through diagnoses, psychiatric problems are addressed as medical problems – and yet they are not just that; (2) Through diagnoses, psychiatric problems are equated with manifest and sometimes transient symptoms – and yet diagnoses have a tendency to reinforce chronicity; (3) Through diagnoses, psychiatric problems appear as "nothing special", because many of us could be diagnosed at any given point in time – and yet normalizing the disorders may cause problems for people if this means that their problems cannot be recognized as sufficiently serious. There are indeed many paradoxes inherent in the logics of diagnostic cultures, which in itself might add to the suffering felt by those who live in these cultures and are diagnosed. Unsurprising, it is easier to explain one's problem to oneself and others if it can be physically observed like a fracture or a tumour.

Expanding Diagnostics

The term "diagnostic cultures" is meant to point to the spread of diagnostic vocabulary and associated social practices to new areas of sociocultural life. But it is also meant to designate more concretely the increasing number of people, who are "living under the description" of a diagnosis (Martin, 2007). Today, we witness a diagnostic expansion in (at least) two ways: In many countries, more and more people receive a psychiatric diagnosis, and new diagnoses are continuously fabricated and suggested, some of which end up entering the official manuals (ICD and DSM), while others stay on the fringes of medical practice. In 1952, when DSM-I appeared, there were 106 diagnostic categories in a manual of 130 pages. In 1994, with DSM-IV, the number of diagnoses had increased to 297 in a manual of 886 pages (Williams, 2009). And now that DSM-5[4] has been published, we see 15 new diagnoses (including hoarding and cannabis withdrawal), and elimination of a few others (most remarkably Asperger's Syndrome). The number of official diagnoses thus increased dramatically in the latter half of the 20th century, but seems now to be slowing down.

In spite of the different changes, Rachel Cooper concludes in her recent book on DSM-5: "The most striking thing about the DSM-5 is how very similar it is to the DSM-IV" (Cooper, 2014, p. 60). This is particularly striking in light of the huge efforts that were put in to discussing and reconstructing the diagnostic system. Originally, the ambition while developing DSM-5 had been to instigate a paradigm shift equivalent to that which occurred in the transition from DSM-II to DSM-III in 1980. The transition in 1980 had implied a change from an etiological approach to diagnosis, with the doctor employing a holistic approach that took the patient's entire biography into account, based in large parts on psychoanalytic theory, to a purely symptom-based approach to diagnosis in DSM-III. Horwitz has simply referred to this transition as one in which etiological psychiatry was replaced by "diagnostic psychiatry" (Horwitz, 2002). After DSM-III a diagnosis was (and is still) made by counting symptoms within a given period of time (e.g. two weeks). The change to DSM-5 was thought to imply a similar shift, only this time away from a categorical approach, where

---

4 Note the change to Arabic numerals, which is thought to facilitate the creation of more editions of the manuals in the future, e.g. DSM-5.1, DSM-5.2 etc.

one either has or does not have a mental disorder based on the number and severity of symptoms, to a dimensional approach, where everyone can be placed somewhere on the continua. But the efforts to construct a dimensional system failed, and instead the chapters of the manual were reorganized. The similarity of the two editions of DSM – number IV and number 5 – means that many of the criticisms that were raised in response to DSM-IV (e.g. by Kutchins & Kirk, 1997) still pertain to DSM-5, and ironically are now voiced by people such as Allen Frances who were centrally placed when DSM-IV was created (Frances, 2013). (Frances was the chair of the DSM-IV task force.)

In addition to the rise in the number of people diagnosed, and also in the number of diagnoses that it is possible to give, there is according to some studies a third kind of rise, *viz.* in the number of people who *ought* to be given a psychiatric diagnosis, but who are currently not diagnosed. This is the problem of under-diagnosis, which co-exists with claims about over-diagnosis. Strictly speaking, these two tendencies can logically occur simultaneously if it is the case that ill people are *not* diagnosed and well people *are* diagnosed. The difference between the number of people who are diagnosed, and the number of people who *ought* to be diagnosed, is called the treatment gap, because a psychiatric diagnosis is in many societal contexts the obligatory passage point to treatment. According to authoritative estimates, the treatment gap for most mental disorders is more than 50 per cent (and for some, such as substance abuse, considerably higher), which means that more than half of those suffering from a mental disorder are not treated (Kohn, Saxena, Levav & Saraceno, 2004). References to the treatment gap can be used by patient organizations, researchers, professionals, and the medical industry to support the view that "more needs to be done" in finding and treating the mentally ill among us. The diagnoses are here central, because they define what mental illness is and how it should be found.

A good example of the discourse of expanding diagnostics can be found on the webpage of the World Health Organization,[5] which states the following:

> Lifetime prevalence rates for any kind of psychological disorder are higher than previously thought, are increasing in recent cohorts and affect nearly half the population.
> Despite being common, mental illness is underdiagnosed by doctors. Less than half of those who meet diagnostic criteria for psychological disorders are identified by doctors.
> Patients, too, appear reluctant to seek professional help. Only 2 in every 5 people experiencing a mood, anxiety or substance use disorder seeking (*sic*) assistance in the year of the onset of the disorder.

This is indeed a very dramatic message: the prevalence rates for *any* psychological disorder are higher than we thought and are rising – now affecting nearly half of us

---

5   http://www.who.int/mental_health/prevention/genderwomen/en/

around the world! The disorders are underdiagnosed (cf. the treatment gap), in part because people do not seek help when they suffer. Seemingly, the prevalence rates are taken at face value, and the WHO does not even consider that one reason why people do not seek help can be because they do not feel they have a psychiatric problem – even when their problem meets the diagnostic criteria for a mental disorder. Needless to say, it can also be the case that people do not receive help, because no help is available (or is too expensive where they live), but the point is that there are likely to be many reasons for not being treated for what is allegedly a mental disorder.

The expanding diagnostics are seen around the world, but this book is almost exclusively about the so-called West, where half of the population is said to be mentally disordered in their lifetime and approximately a quarter of the population within any one year (Wittchen & Jacobi, 2005). In the West there are certain, quite fixed, ideas about what counts as mental disorder, as specified in the diagnostic manuals, and although the DSM (in particular) affects the local understandings of mental problems all over the world (Watters, 2010), there are still curious differences and exceptions. One such exception was reported in June 2014 in Nigeria, when Mubarak Bala was sent for psychiatric treatment because of a case of *atheism*. His disbelief in God was here interpreted as a mental disorder, likely an effect of schizophrenia, and he was detained against his will in a psychiatric ward. Fortunately, he has since been released, but is allegedly living in danger because of his (dis-)beliefs that were pathologized by the local doctors.[6] This extreme example illustrates the variability in what counts as mental disorder and how psychiatry and larger cultural and political issues are intertwined. This is easy to see for Westerners when finding an extreme case in Nigeria, but it is much harder to notice in our own diagnostic cultures, given the way that the current conceptualizations of mental disorder are being naturalized through the diagnostic categories. That is to say, it has become hard for us Westerners to think of mental disorder outside what is made possible by the psychiatric categories. This means that the psychiatric-diagnostic discourse is close to becoming hegemonic, and even those who are aware of the negative effects of diagnosis – who argue, to quote Rachel Cooper, that diagnosis "suggests that the source of a problem should be located within an individual, and [...] tends to remove an issue from the political or ethical domain" (Cooper, 2014, p. 4) – often remain caught in a diagnostic language when addressing the problems raised by diagnostics: does the pathologization of sadness make us depressed, for example?

At this point I hope I have provided enough examples to indicate what I mean in this book when addressing the *diagnostic cultures* of contemporary society. It is important to use the term cultures in the plural, because there is not a monolithic, agreed-upon understanding of mental disorder delivered by the diagnoses, and there is no unitary way that the diagnostic language is used. Diagnostic categories are used in numerous ways, by sufferers, parents, teachers, managers,

---

6   See http://iheu.org/mubarak-bala-is-free/.

clinicians, medical doctors, psychiatrists, psychologists, researchers, policy makers, social workers etc., and, within these different groups, there is also much heterogeneity concerning diagnostics: there are patient groups that fight *for* the right to be diagnosed (recognized) and others that fight *against* being diagnosed (pathologized). How can one determine what in one case is a proper recognition of suffering through a diagnosis and what in another case represents illegitimate pathologization of deviant or eccentric behaviours? This is not an easy task, and not something this book can settle once and for all. Instead, the task will be to unfold the societal situation through the concept of diagnostic cultures, charting some of the ways in which diagnoses operate in people's personal lives and on a larger social scale.

Nikolas Rose has recently summed up the societal functions of diagnoses in (what I call) our diagnostic cultures (adapted from Rose, 2013), illustrating the huge variability in how diagnoses work:

1. A diagnosis is a condition of suitability of an individual for treatment – without a diagnosis of pathology, there is generally no case for treating the person.
2. In insurance based regimes, it is a condition of financial coverage of the cost of treatment.
3. For those who are employed, it can be a condition of legitimate absence from work.
4. For those who are unemployed, it may be a condition for access to welfare benefits.
5. For hospitals and medical establishments it is a central feature of patient records, which often shape the allocation of funding from those who commission services for various conditions.
6. For lawyers, it can be a condition for involuntary detention and treatment.
7. In the school system, a diagnosis may be the basis of allocation to special educational provision.
8. For epidemiologists, diagnostic categories are the very basis of their estimates and predictions that are based on assessments of incidence and prevalence.
9. For planners of services, those estimates and predictions are the essential raw materials for their work.
10. For funders of research, especially charities focused on a particular disorder, diagnoses may delineate a problem that is really worthy of investigation.

The list could have been considerably longer, so although psychiatric diagnoses were created as the work tools of psychiatrists, we see that they today operate in and between a large number of social practices, in addition to providing the individual with an experience of getting an explanation for his or her problems. Diagnoses affect how people feel and interpret themselves, they enter different social arenas (in schools, at work and at home) and are used to regulate a huge number of practices, and they have complex histories leading up to how they are used today. So where can one find an analytic framework that enables one to study the phenomenological, discursive, and historical aspects of a phenomenon such as diagnoses? My answer in this book points to cultural psychology to which I will now turn. Readers who are familiar with this theoretical paradigm may jump directly to the next chapter, and others, who find the theoretical framework overly abstract, may also read the more content rich chapters first before returning to the theory unfolded in the rest of this first chapter.

Cultural Psychology

Cultural psychology has a long history, going back quite directly to the work of Lev Vygotsky in Russia in the early 20th century (Vygotsky, 1978), and more indirectly to different philosophical bases. Vygotsky drew inspiration from many sources, but was placed in the tradition of Marxism, trying to address the relationships between mind and world, individual and society, dialectically rather than as separate entities that somehow interact. One can trace this line of thought back in time to philosophers such as Hegel and Spinoza, and it stands in contrast to Cartesian dualist philosophies, depicting subject and object as discrete entities. This is not the place to unfold a full history of cultural psychology; others have done this much more thoroughly, for example Jaan Valsiner and Rene van der Veer (2000). In their book, they trace the notion of the *social* mind, which was found not just in the work of Vygotsky, but also in that of American pragmatists such as John Dewey and George Herbert Mead. The dialectical approach offers the idea that the mind is social, and that the social is also "minded". In other words, as Valsiner puts it: "Human beings are *individually social* and *socially individual*." (Valsiner, 2014, p. 53). It is simply not possible to delineate two different ontological realms, one of minds of individuals, and another of culture or "the social". Instead, persons – human beings considered as creatures with minds and not simply as physiological organisms – belong to culture, and culture belongs to persons (Valsiner, 2007, p. 21). This means that psychology, sociology and anthropology are all needed to create the discipline of cultural psychology, and other disciplines could and should be added, in particular history, because cultural psychology sees every mental/cultural process as existing and developing in historical time. There is a focus on culture as a historical *process* rather than an entity or substance. Culture is not a thing, and, for cultural psychologists, it has no agentive or causal powers (Valsiner, 2014). Thus, culture does not *do* anything; culture does not act and culture does not cause *us* to act either. Culture is not a variable that can be isolated and measured. "How much of our active life is determined by culture?" is a meaningless question from this perspective, because culture does not determine anything, and it would not be possible to calculate its relative importance (alongside biology, nature or genes, for example) anyway. It would be more correct to say that everything in the human world is cultural – just as everything in the human world is natural (mainly because it is natural for humans to live as cultural beings).

From the point of view of cultural psychology, only *persons* (not culture) act (Brinkmann, 2011b). Unlike other psychological approaches that approach mental phenomena as aspects of a *mind*, or neuroscientific approaches that view them as aspects of a brain, cultural psychologists argue that psychological predicates pertain to persons only. They are neither "mindists" or "brainists" but "personists" (Sprague, 1999). This also separates cultural psychologists from many sociologists who operate with social structures or entities as having some sort of agentive power. Only persons have this kind of power, but no human action would be possible without culture. So, even though culture is not a variable, a force or an agent, it is *everywhere* in human life and minds. Culture is a name for all those *mediators* that *persons* use when performing actions, thinking thoughts or feeling emotions. Language, for example, is a cultural tool that mediates the human capacity for conceptual thought and enables complex forms of communication and self-consciousness. Language is particularly important for cultural psychologists because it is what enables human beings to create a distance to the here-and-now contexts that they are in. The process of creating distance – and reflecting upon the context, one's preferences and desires to act – is called *semiotic mediation* by cultural psychologists (Valsiner, 2007, p. 33). Sign *mediators* such as language are not exactly the same as *means*. For means quite directly enable one to realize one's pre-formed intentions (means-ends reasoning), whereas mediators at once constitute and transform the intentions that they carry. When we think abstract thoughts, for example, it is not the case that we have pre-linguistic ideas that we somehow translate into language that we can communicate to others. Rather, it is the case that we use language to think the very thoughts that we have. Language is, as Wittgenstein said, "the vehicle of thought" (Wittgenstein, 1953, § 329). In this sense, language mediates the activity of thinking, and the categories we use in thinking mediate the actions we may undertake. I cannot celebrate Christmas, for example, without the category "Christmas", but this does not mean that Christmas is a purely linguistic or discursive event. Obviously, Christmas is a set of *practices*, which involve semiotic *and* material tools, ranging from trees and presents to carols and holidays and many other things that have evolved historically. To return to the notion of agency: cultural psychologists will argue (the quite obvious point) that *persons* celebrate Christmas. It is not the tree or the presents that celebrate this event; rather, persons are the irreducible agents in cultural life (Harré, 1983). However, it is equally obvious that persons could not celebrate Christmas, or even have the intentions to do so, without a whole range of mediators, some of which are semiotic while others are material, both of which are equally important in constituting the *practices* of Christmas.

Now, the ambition in this book is not to study Christmas cultures. Other cultural psychologists could do this, and it would be a fascinating topic. The ambition is to study diagnostic cultures, and the complexities already introduced –

of persons and practices, semiosis[7] and materialities, all in dialectical relationships – necessitate a comprehensive and yet precise framework of cultural psychology. The various schools and traditions within cultural psychology put emphasis on slightly different aspects of minded-persons-in-practices, and I find that they are all legitimate and fruitful for the project of this book. This is why I will turn to briefly unfold three aspects of sociocultural life studied by cultural psychologists, but first I shall say a little bit more about the concept of *mind*, which is just as important as *culture* for cultural psychologists.

What is the Mind?

In the version of cultural psychology articulated here, the mind is conceived as normative (Brinkmann, 2006; see also Brinkmann, 2011b, on which the following is based). This has significant consequences for the analyses of what we think of as mental *disorders*, as we shall see particularly in Chapter 7. That the mind is normative means that the mind cannot be equated with purely receptive or experiential consciousness, or what is sometimes referred to as qualia in contemporary philosophy of mind; nor can it be equated with any substance or entity, not even the material entity of the brain. Why is that? Because if the mind were identical with some causally operating process or entity in the world or brain, we could have no way of distinguishing psychological phenomena from physiological ones, and since we are in fact able to make this distinction, it means that the mind cannot be purely causal. An example from Harré (1983) may illustrate what this means: although dread, anger, indigestion and exhaustion all have behavioural manifestations as well as fairly distinctive experiential qualities (qualia), we have no trouble concluding that only the two former phenomena should be included among psychological (or mental) phenomena, whereas the latter two are physiological. Why so? Because, argues Harré, dread and anger are psychological phenomena to the extent that they fall within a normative moral order, where they can be evaluated according to local norms of correctness and appropriateness. Dread and anger do not merely happen, like physiological phenomena, but are *done* (by skilful human persons), and are therefore subject to normative and indeed moral appraisal. One can feel and express legitimate as well as illegitimate anger, whereas indigestion may be painful and annoying, but it is meaningless to say that it can be legitimate or the opposite. Mental phenomena – our ways of perceiving, acting, remembering and feeling – do not simply happen, but can be done more or less well relative to cultural customs, norms and conventions. In short, they are normative.

To study the mind is thus to study a set of skills and dispositions to act, feel and think in particular ways, and we cannot determine whether someone has a skill by examining the person's brain, but only by studying the acting person in her practical life activities. To have a mind is not to have some "thing" attached to the

---

7   Processes involving the use of signs.

brain or the body (for skills are not "things"); rather, for a creature to have a mind "is for it to have a distinctive range of capacities of intellect and will, in particular the conceptual capacities of a language-user which make self-awareness and self-reflection possible" (Bennett & Hacker, 2003, p. 105). In other words, using the concept of mind is to use "a generic term for our various abilities, dispositions and their relationships" (Coulter, 1979, p. 13). It is not to talk about a place (e.g. the "inner world") or an object (e.g. the brain). Hilary Putnam has made a similar point from the standpoint of pragmatism: "the mind is not a thing; talk of our minds is to talk of world-involving capabilities that we have and capacities that we engage in" (Putnam, 1999, pp. 169–170). As we shall see in this book, this has consequences for how we should address mental disorders as one species of mental phenomena of persons.

Cultural psychologists reject the widespread tendency in psychology and our culture as a whole to reify the mind by treating it as an independent entity, which "does" certain things (attends, remembers etc.). The mind does not do these things, just as culture does not do anything. Only *persons* do such things, and it is exactly their capacities, abilities, capabilities and dispositions to do these things that we refer to with the term "mind". Valsiner (2007, p. 125) refers to a related fallacy as "entification", which is the fallacy of treating psychological constructs (e.g. personality, intelligence *or* mental disorders) as causal entities "in the mind" that cause persons to do certain things. Again, it is better to follow the pragmatist John Dewey and insist that psychological phenomena are adverbial (see Brinkmann, 2013a); they concern things done, which means that there are no psychological *entities* as such (e.g. intelligence, anger, depression), but only persons and what they do (and they may indeed act intelligently, angrily, depressed etc.). (See also Billig, 1999, for a convincing defence of an adverbial approach to the emotions.)

Thus, cultural psychologists insist that it is fruitful to think of the mind as a verb rather than a noun, as an activity or process rather than a static entity, and, when we do so, we address the mind as a normative phenomenon: as a set of skills and dispositions to act, think and feel. With this framework some old problems dissolve and new ones arise. The Cartesian problem of how to find a place for the mind in a physical universe is no longer pertinent, for this problem presupposed that the mind was an (immaterial) substance that somehow had to be hooked up with the material world. If the mind is not a substance, though, it is neither material nor immaterial. Skills and dispositions are hardly approachable in these terms. (A question such as: "Are the golfing skills of Tiger Woods material or immaterial?" sounds mysterious to say the least, for skills cut across such strange divides.) Instead, the question to ask is what enables the skills and dispositions to unfold and come under control of persons. The answer given by cultural psychology – at least in the version advocated here – is that *mediators* constitute and enable the skills and dispositions of people. So, there is an inner conceptual connection between *persons*, *minds*, *culture* and *mediators*.

Elsewhere I have suggested that four sets of mediators are particularly important in this regard (Brinkmann, 2011b): brain, body, practices and technologies. These are generic sets of mediators, and it may sound strange to talk about the brain, for example, as a mediator of mental life, but what it means is quite simple: the brain can be thought of as a tool that mediates human life activities. Humans use their brains when performing the cultural tasks that make up a life (Harré & Moghaddam, 2012), and when the brain does not function adequately, say, if someone begins to suffer from dementia, then it is sometimes possible to use auxiliary devices such as Post-it notes with names written on them, if the person cannot recall the names of things simply by using the brain. This illustrates how technology (in a broad sense, including Post-it notes) can serve a psychological function. In the same way, our bodies and the social practices in which we participate mediate the ways we perform the tasks of psychological life. I will return to this later in the book (Chapter 7), when I seek to develop a cultural psychological understanding of mental disorder, which builds on the idea that "disorder" can have many different sources in brains, bodies, practices and material culture, and which identifies the important roles played by our conceptual designations (e.g. through diagnoses).

Three Aspects of Sociocultural Life

This whole complex of acting, embodied persons in a sociomaterial world (who may experience problems that can be diagnosed) has been studied from different perspectives by different cultural psychologists. It is unsurprising that scholars have needed to purify certain perspectives and downplay others, given the complexity at hand. At least three distinct approaches can be singled out, which are all important to the analyses of the present book. They are depicted below in Figure 1.1.

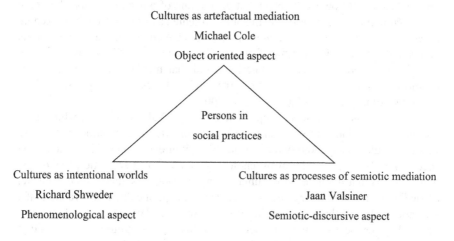

Figure 1.1   Three aspects of sociocultural life

In the middle we have what most cultural psychologists agree on studying: acting persons involved in social practice. We study not brains or information processing apparatuses, but living, suffering, acting, feeling, thinking persons. They – or we – can, however, only act in social practices. Celebrating Christmas is only celebrating Christmas because of the social practices of this event and their histories. Absent the historically developed practices of Christmas, and dancing around the tree would be nothing but meaningless twists and jerks. Social practices, however, are not static, but are constantly and creatively renewed and restructured. Around the centre, we have three schools, or traditions, of cultural psychology, which share many premises, but which have slightly different emphases and approach acting persons from different perspectives.

We have the school represented by Richard Shweder (1990), who argues that cultural psychology studies what he calls "intentional worlds", which are sociocultural environments that are constituted by the representations and interpretations that human beings direct at it. Intentional worlds can usefully be studied using phenomenological approaches; that is, approaches that take an interest in the life world of human beings, how they experience and act in the world prior to formulating explicit theories (e.g. scientific theories) about it. In relation to diagnostic cultures, the phenomenological aspects concern how people experience the process of being diagnosed and how diagnoses appear in their lived experience.

Next, we have the school represented by Michael Cole (2003), whose cultural psychology is a kind of activity theory or cultural historical theory. Coming from a Marxist perspective, the key idea here is that human activity is mediated by different material artefacts. Our relationship to the social and material world is mediated by everything from shovels to computers. In relation to diagnostic cultures, it is the case that diagnoses themselves can be conceived of as epistemic objects (see the following chapter) that gain a kind of objective status when they come to function in the world, and the object oriented aspects obviously also come in when we look at how these diagnostic cultures are co-constituted by numerous things and technologies, ranging from standardized tests and databases, to pills and clinics. There is an entire material world that mediates the emergence of diagnostic cultures – or, one could say that such cultures are partly "assembled" by a range of material mediators (Latour, 2005).

Finally, we have the school represented by Jaan Valsiner (2014), which does not deny the importance of intentional worlds or artefact-mediation, but whose version of cultural psychology focuses our analytic attention on *semiotic* mediation specifically. Valsiner's cultural psychology is a version of semiotic psychology, which means that it studies how human beings use signs, symbols, language etc. as mediators in and of their lives together. The concept of culture here refers to the semiotic mediation that is part of the system of organized psychological functions. From this perspective, persons necessarily belong to culture – yet, culture necessarily belongs to persons. In relation to diagnostic cultures, it is quite evident that psychiatric diagnoses have a significant role to play as semiotic mediators that are put to use by individuals and collectives to regulate a large number of processes in modern society.

The three aspects focus on different approaches to cultural psychology, but the view in this book is that they do not exclude each other; rather they provide a more complete picture if put together. Contemporary diagnostic cultures have an *experienced* aspect, since they are populated by living, sensing human beings who often understand their problems in light of the diagnostic categories they are offered by medical and psychological authorities. They also have an *object* aspect with the many material mediators that play a role, and they certainly have a *semiotic* aspect, which, in other traditions, is studied as *discourses* (Gee, 2005) or *social representations* (Schmitz, Filippone & Edelman, 2003). Each is an aspect of a cultural whole, and each aspect is influenced by the others in ways that cannot be predicted until one looks closely at the empirical world. Diagnoses have a cultural history (as objects) and affect the ways in which people experience their lives (phenomenology) and the ways they talk reflectively about their problems (semiosis). As we shall see in Chapter 3, these are all aspects of social practices, which represent the core of cultural life: acting persons in social practices.

All aspects, as I see them, are infused with *normativity*, as I argued above, and what is interesting in relation to psychiatric diagnoses and mental disorders is that normativity becomes particularly problematic. Do persons really *do* OCD, depression, ADHD etc. relative to cultural norms, or do these afflictions *happen* to them? One significant conclusion of the present book (shared, for example, with Martin, 2007) is that people in fact *do* their disorders through diagnoses, although rarely in a fully explicit and willed manner. People *do* ADHD, but they also *have* it, and might even come to think of themselves as *being* ADHD. These three dimensions (which will be unpacked more thoroughly in the following chapter) correspond in some ways to the aspects studied by cultural psychologists: the phenomenological aspect is primarily about how people experience their lives *as* suffering from a disorder. Thus, a phenomenological approach is useful when one is interested in the self-identity of the diagnosed. The object aspect is about what people say (using a diagnostic category) they have, when they *have* a mental disorder. The diagnosis itself can here be studied as an object in the world with a biography (Daston & Galison, 2007). Finally, people also *perform* or do their disorders through the diagnoses, which points to a discursive or semiotic aspect that stresses the performative nature of mental life. All aspects of sociocultural life are affected by today's diagnostic cultures – or so I hope to demonstrate and discuss in the following pages.

Critiques of Psychiatry

Before moving on to the next chapter, I shall here return to the discussion of psychiatry and diagnoses, by summarizing four of the most important critiques that have been directed at psychiatric ideas, several of which will play important roles in the remainder of this book (and are helpfully articulated by Busfield, 2011). By referring to these critiques, I hope to show that the discussion of diagnoses plays a role in all of them, albeit in different ways.

(1) The first states that psychiatry is inhumane and ineffective, which is a classic critique that was articulated, for example, by Erving Goffman (1961) in a famous study of life in a psychiatric hospital. After the emergence of anti-psychiatric movements in the 1960s and 1970s (represented by Ronald Laing, Thomas Szasz and Goffman himself), much has changed in psychiatry, but the classic critique has nonetheless been rearticulated in recent years with a focus on the dangers of psychopharmacology and the use of force in psychiatric hospitals. Well-known international critical voices are represented by Robert Whitaker (2010) and David Healy (2012), who have argued that the so-called iatrogenic effects (the disease producing effects) of long-term use of psychiatric drugs are so massive that they often outweigh the possible benefits of using the drugs. This conclusion is currently hotly debated, which testifies to the enduring relevance of this kind of critique. I return to this point below, most thoroughly in Chapter 6, where I present some interpretations of the current epidemics of mental disorders, some of which might be related to the harmful effects of drugs. Since diagnoses represent the gateway to treatment, they are at least indirectly struck by this first line of criticism.

(2) The second major critique states that psychiatry's categorical model of psychopathology is faulty. Unlike Freud's dimensional approach to mental disorder, according to which everyone is to be found somewhere on the psychopathological dimensions and axes (which means that we all, in a way, have a grain of each of the mental disorders), current diagnostic practices are built upon the idea of disease specificity, which implies that the mental disorders can in principle be clearly delineated from each other, so that one either has them or does not have them. As recounted above, when DSM-5 was developed, some commentators hoped that it would change into a dimensional model, but it ended up building on the same categorical approach as previous editions of the manual (Cooper, 2014). After Freud, it was especially Hans Eysenck who became famous for a dimensional personality theory (according to which an individual personality can be understood through the dimensions neuroticism, psychoticism and introversion/extroversion), and who criticized psychiatry's conception of disorder for its lack of dimensionality. In the next chapter, I return to the notion of disease specificity and its relationship to diagnoses.

(3) A third group of researchers, most of them belonging to the anti-psychiatric movement, have radicalized the critique of the categorical model of psychopathology and argued that it is misguided in the first place to even have a concept of mental illness. Thomas Szasz is the best known of these critics, who from the 1960s attacked what he called "the myth of mental illness" (Szasz, 1961). His critique is grounded in an argument that the concept of illness rightly belongs to somatic medicine, since it logically refers to lesions and dysfunctions

in organs and other forms of bodily tissue. Szasz argued that instead of talking of mental illness, we should approach mental disorders as "problems in living". If not, we simply stigmatize human suffering and deviation as pathological, and thus medicalize and pathologize life, something that was particularly evident in the Soviet Union, for example, when political dissidents were treated as mentally ill. Pathologization will be a key theme throughout the book.

Partly as a reaction to the anti-psychiatric critique, it has become common to talk about mental *disorder* rather than illness, but, in principle, the challenge for psychiatrists remains the same regardless of the terminology: that of identifying *what it is* that is disordered or ill, if it is not just (as Szasz would argue) the individual's way of life as such. For if it is uniquely a person's actions that are perceived as problematic (either by the person or by people around him or her), then it seems reasonable to address these as problems in living that we rightly judge in moral or legal terms. Discourses of illness or disorder seem to presuppose a more clearly defined physical object that can be damaged and which calls for medical judgment and intervention.

In recent decades, many researchers in the biomedical sciences have pinned their hopes on the possibility that neuroscience can identify mental disorders with a damaged object, *viz.* the brain (or parts of it), but so far no valid biomarkers have been found in psychiatry that would make possible a diagnostic process using a brain scan (Singh & Rose, 2009). Singh and Rose demonstrate that the widespread idea that it is possible to diagnose psychiatric disorders through genetic screening or brain scanning is wrong, and the hunt for biomarkers, which goes on in many corners of the biomedical sciences, represents a remarkable shift in psychiatry away from concentrating on identifying the causes of suffering (in ontogenesis or social life) and to charting the physical correlates of experienced suffering. (See also Rose & Abi-Rached, 2013, who provide a thorough discussion of the role of the neurosciences in this regard.) There is much that indicates that the hunt for simple, determining biomarkers is futile, since both the neurological and genetic backgrounds to mental disorders are at once much more complex, heterogeneous and particularistic than previously assumed. Singh and Rose conclude that information from biomarkers alone is insufficient to explain most of the variance in observed behaviors (Singh & Rose, 2009, p. 205).

The most thoroughly worked-out attempt in recent years to conceptualize the "psychiatric object", which may be ill or disordered, is that of Jerome Wakefield (1992). His theory of mental illness is called the "harmful dysfunction" theory, since it has these two components. In order for us to talk about mental illness, Wakefield states, there should first be something that is *harmful*. A person can only be said to be mentally ill, if that person experiences suffering or distress to some extent. Wakefield explains how this first component is a value component, since he believes that social norms and values determine the extent to which something counts as suffering or distress. How much one should suffer in order for the suffering to be pathological varies across epochs and cultures. Besides this value component, there is also a purely factual component stemming from a *dysfunction*, he claims. One is not mentally ill, just because one suffers, since suffering can be caused by all kinds of problems and life situations. Only if the suffering is related to a dysfunction in the person's mental processes can the person rightly be said to be mentally ill (or disordered).

Wakefield here mobilizes arguments from evolutionary psychology, where researchers invoke the existence of genetically based "mental modules" to account for mental functioning. Mental modules are said to be innate psychobiological mechanisms analogous to physiological mechanisms in bodily organs. Just as a heart can be dysfunctional, when something is wrong with it that makes it unable to operate adequately as a blood pump, so a mental module can be dysfunctional if it, say, causes a person to feel constant fear without any frightening object being present. It is not pathological to feel fear if one is a soldier who is about to attack the enemy, but if a similar kind of fear is felt in everyday situations that are objectively safe *and* if the discomfort is caused by defective mental modules, then we are entitled (says Wakefield) to talk about mental illness. The object that may "break" and become dysfunctional (and thus produce mental illness) is thus a mental module. In short, for Wakefield, a mental dysfunction is a failure of the capacity of a mental mechanism to perform a function for which it was biologically designed. I return to this theory in Chapter 7.

(4) This takes us directly to the fourth influential critique of psychiatry, which is also in focus in the present book: that diagnoses pathologize. A consequence of Wakefield's two-component theory is that quite a few of psychiatry's existing diagnoses must be said to be pathologizing by implicitly breaking down the distinction between life problems and psychopathology. Together with Allan Horwitz, a medical sociologist, Wakefield has thus argued that the diagnostic criteria for depression (Horwitz & Wakefield, 2007) and anxiety (Horwitz & Wakefield, 2012) are overinclusive and do not make possible a necessary distinction between common sadness and clinical depression, or between normal fear and pathological anxiety. The main reason is that the component of dysfunction has not been developed in psychiatric diagnostics. A diagnosis is formulated by psychiatrists by examining the symptoms, and counting them using checklists, and it is therefore much more difficult to assess whether the symptoms are caused by an underlying mental dysfunction or rather by a given life situation. Significant sadness, Wakefield and Horwitz maintain, should only be diagnosed as depression if there is a dysfunction involved (and not just if the person has been divorced or has suffered a loss, for example), but the existing diagnostic category does not capture this difference adequately.

Wakefield's theory of mental disorder as harmful dysfunction thus holds significant critical potential, yet without being anti-psychiatric or rejecting the concept of mental illness as such. It can serve to warn researchers and practitioners in the psychiatric fields of illegitimate pathologizations of ordinary (harmful) experiences and conditions, which are not dysfunctional (and therefore not expressions of mental disorders). The main problem related to pathologization is that unpleasant experiences and conditions may be related to various social problems such as marginalization, poverty and social injustice, which run the risk of being interpreted as individual psychopathology when looked upon through the diagnostic lens – and when the authoritative understanding of some experience or problem employs the psychiatric interpretation (and approaches something as, say, depression), it is of course natural to act as if it is a psychiatric problem (and treat it with anti-depressants, for instance). To repeat a basic point: the risk is that pathologizing something leads to an individualization of social problems and narrows down our ways of understanding and treating the problems that people have (Brinkmann, 2014a).

However, there are also certain problems inherent in Wakefield's theory, and it has often been criticized (e.g. Bolton, 2008). Perhaps its most significant problem is its lack of specification concerning what mental modules are. The theory rests on the premise that there are such mental modules, developed in the course of natural history to solve specific problems in humanity's evolutionary childhood, and that these modules are innate and relatively independent of sociocultural contexts, but critics of Wakefield here (rightly, in my view) object that this represents an outdated view of the nature-nurture relationship (in this case, the relationship between mental modules and social practices), which presents them as different and perhaps contradictory forces. Many contemporary researchers in biology (e.g. Sterelny, 2012) and anthropology (e.g. Ingold, 2011) now reject the idea that we can separate what is psychobiologically innate from what is acquired socioculturally.

Human psychology, including the sufferings of human beings, is most likely always biological and sociocultural in a way that makes it impossible to draw a firm distinction between these as separate components. In the words of Lock and Nguyen: "culture, history, politics, and biology (environmental and individual) are inextricably entangled and subject to never-ending transformations [...] biological and social life is mutually constitutive" (Lock & Nguyen, 2010, p. 1). This leads these authors to an intriguing concept of "local biologies", that Lock has worked on for several years (Lock, 2001). Such recent ideas of entanglements of the biological and the cultural suggest that the very idea of innate mental modules may be a myth, or at least too speculative to serve as the basis for a theory of mental disorder. I shall not pursue this argument further here (I return to it later in the book), but just conclude that even if Wakefield's theory has considerable problems regarding its positive definition of mental disorder, it nonetheless offers a very significant critique of many existing psychiatric diagnoses, since it highlights the widespread confusion of ordinary, painful phenomena of life with mental disorders. I believe there is much to learn from Wakefield's critique of the pathologizing effects of some diagnoses without having to accept his theory of mental disorder as such – and there is likewise much to learn from scholars who break down the distinction between the biological and the sociocultural in relation to mental disorders.

The four lines of criticism mentioned here – (1) that psychiatry is inhumane, (2) that the categorical model is faulty, (3) that the very idea of mental illness is misconstrued, and (4) that the diagnoses, or at least some of them, are pathologizing – are important as a background to discussions of the notion of mental disorder and of the relationship between diagnoses and disorders, which will be central themes throughout this book.

Chapter 2
Psychiatric Diagnoses as Epistemic Objects

Diagnoses are classifications of diseases, illnesses or disorders. The word comes from the Greek term for distinction or assessment. *Dia* literally means through or via, and *gnosis* is knowledge. So a diagnosis is something through which we may gain knowledge of diseases. A diagnosis should enable us to distinguish between various abnormal conditions. The English term first appeared in 1681, and the project of developing disease classifications took off in the 18th century, when different sciences in general became obsessed with categorizing and measuring many different properties of the world (Jutel, 2011, p. 6). According to the historian of medicine Charles Rosenberg, the more recent history of medical diagnoses is closely connected to what he calls disease specificity. This refers to the modern idea that diseases are specific entities that have a kind of independent existence beyond their unique manifestations in sick individuals (Rosenberg, 2007, p. 13). The idea of disease specificity is so ingrained in medical practices today, and has become quite obvious for patients and professionals alike, that it is difficult to imagine that it was once different. But, according to Rosenberg's studies, this was in fact once different. Disease specificity is a cultural idea from the end of the 19th century that has enabled people since to imagine diseases as discrete conditions in an organism, which can be defined and separated relatively clearly from other diseases, and which are therefore identical with similar conditions in other organisms. Needless to say, this applies to somatic medicine, where examples such as cancer or diabetes can serve as illustrations, but it has also become a commonplace in psychiatry, although the idea is here more debatable, as we shall see in this chapter.

The idea of disease specificity has been established in psychiatry through the dissemination of diagnostic categories in DSM (the classification system of the American Psychiatric Association) and ICD (the WHO's system), particularly since the middle of the 20th century. When a category exists (such as ADHD, OCD or PTSD), it is easily taken as a matter of course that it refers to real, existing objects in the world. The idea that the diagnoses point to objectively existing instances of universal forms of mental disorder has been generally accepted in our diagnostic cultures. However, as Frances has critically pointed out: "Billions of research dollars have failed to produce convincing evidence that any mental disorder is a discrete disease entity with a unitary cause." (Frances, 2013, p. 19), while Rosenberg demonstrates that the relationship between diagnoses (categories) and disorders (forms of suffering) is extremely complex: "Diagnosis labels, defines, and predicts, and, in doing so, helps constitute and legitimate the reality that it discerns" (Rosenberg, 2007, p. 16). The formulation of diagnoses in a society leads to a naturalization and legitimation of different problematic conditions and forms of suffering, given that they become linked to a system of practices that handles these conditions. Critics often refer to this as a medicalization of deviance, by which different normative breaches are interpreted within a medical framework. Even in those cases (which abound in psychiatry) where an underlying biological component has not been identified, as in ADHD, for example, the diagnosis can help delineate a space of possible suffering, because it establishes an object that one may "have" or not. One may thus "have" ADHD, depression or anxiety. This is made discursively possible through the formulation of a diagnostic category that objectifies the given kind of suffering. This can involve a distinct "entification" (Valsiner, 2007), where the person may experience a concrete "thing within", to which the diagnosis refers (see Chapter 4). And it also becomes possible to *be* hyperactive, depressed or anxious, which refers to an identity dimension associated with the diagnoses. This can be transient (as in the statement "I am depressed today") or chronic (as in: "I'm an Aspie"; that is, someone diagnosed with Asperger's). Finally, one may also *do* or perform something hyperactively, depressively or anxiously, which can be referred to as an adverbial dimension of suffering and mental life in general, having to do with the ways in which things are done.

Building on these three dimensions (having, being, doing) that are enabled by diagnostic categories, I shall in this chapter throw light on psychiatric diagnoses as objects of knowledge. Are genuine mental disorders pre-existing objects that one may simply acquire or not, in relative independence of diagnostic categories? Or could it be that disorders emerge in the world together with the diagnostic categories that point them out? Are we forced to choose between essentialism (the view that diagnoses refer to pre-existing, disease specific objects) and social constructionism (the idea that diagnoses unilaterally construct diseases and disorders)? Or can we articulate a third possibility? How one answers these questions depends on one's conception of diagnoses as *epistemic objects*; that is, as objects of scientific knowledge and intervention (Danziger, 2003).

Having unfolded the three dimensions of mental disorder (having, being, doing), and illustrated how diagnostic categories may affect each of these, I shall introduce the groundbreaking ideas of Ian Hacking on human kinds and begin to articulate the contours of an emerging concept of psychiatric disorder, based on cultural psychology, which may strike a balance between essentialism and social constructionism, and this is continued in later chapters of this book. Finally, I will present a sociological account of how something becomes a psychiatric disorder and what role diagnostics may play in this process.

Having, Being and Doing Mental Disorders: Three Aspects of an Epistemic Object

What do diagnoses make possible in the lives of the diagnosed? The answer I shall give is that they make possible having, being and doing a whole number of things. This can be understood through the concept of the epistemic object. The historian of psychology Kurt Danziger has developed an analysis of psychological phenomena as epistemic objects (Danziger, 2003), and this analysis can be broadened to psychiatry as well. Epistemic objects are the entities that scientists work with and seek to create knowledge about. In psychiatry and psychology some of the epistemic objects are referred to with diagnostic labels (depression, anxiety, ADHD etc.). Epistemic objects can be discursive in the sense that they only exist when they are conceptualized linguistically. This might be the case for Santa Claus, who can only be an object of knowledge, because we have a Santa Claus discourse. But Danziger claims that epistemic objects in psychology also have an extra-discursive or material dimension. This means that they arise as elements in social practices, where humans engage in joint action and coordinate different courses of conduct using a range of technological and material artefacts. Social practices develop historically, and Danziger argues that there are no objects in psychology that are ahistorical. Psychology is here different from physics, because physicists can more or less approach the world as they find it (of course how they find it depends on cultural pre-understandings), but psychologists and psychiatrists constantly create new domains of phenomena, which are constituted by the procedures that produce them.

This may sound mysterious, but Danziger has conducted quite concrete historical studies of a large number of epistemic objects in psychology such as intelligence, behaviour, motivation, personality and attitudes (Danziger, 1997), and, in a classic in the field of the history of psychology, he has demonstrated how the subject psychologists study (that is, the way of being human approached by psychologists) is in many ways an artefact of the experimental procedures that are employed in psychological practices of inquiry (Danziger, 1990). In order for epistemic objects to emerge in the psy-sciences (psychology, psychiatry, psychoanalysis, psychotherapy etc.), three conditions must be in place: first, there must be human beings who are interested in getting to know human phenomena such as forms of suffering; second, there must be social practices; that it, historically developed forms of coordinated action that are meant to solve various problems; and third, there must be instruments that allow for description or measurement of the epistemic objects, such as diagnostic tests.

In what follows we shall take a closer look at diagnoses as epistemic objects. In order to underline what I take to be a fact – that they necessarily operate as elements within social practices – I have placed the person participating in social practice in the middle of the model below. It is important to bear in mind the point that I emphasized in the previous chapter that it is not brains or bodies that suffer and are diagnosed, but rather persons who participate in various life situations conceptualized as social practices. When one experiences a problem (such as a lack of concentration or energy) in the practices of which one is a part, and when such a problem is categorized diagnostically (say, as ADHD or clinical depression), it is relevant to address three aspects of the experienced suffering, which I here call the having, doing and being aspects.

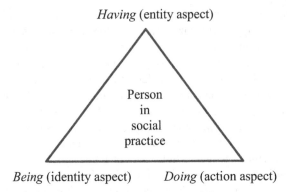

Being (identity aspect)   *Doing* (action aspect)

Figure 2.1   Problems in social practices – having, doing and being aspects

The model is a heuristic model that is meant to be used in qualitative studies of the lives of people with mental problems and diagnoses. It is not meant to be exhaustive of what there is to say on the subject, but is rather conceived as a tool to think with. Beginning with "having" at the top, referring to the entity aspect, we find that this is in clear continuation of the discussion of diagnoses as epistemic objects. Diagnoses can be seen to refer to objects that one may have or not (just as one may wear a hat or not) and we conventionally talk about people who "have" ADHD and other mental disorders, but we very rarely stop and consider what this way of talking implies. When we talk about somatic illness, the entity aspect is more straightforward: one may have a fracture, a malfunctioning heart valve or a malign tumor, for example. But what does it mean to "have" a mental disorder? The simple answer is that one has a mental disorder when one meets the criteria as specified in the reigning diagnostic manuals. Obviously, this simply moves the problem one step back, because we then need to know what it means to "have" the conditions specified in the manuals. DSM-5 defines a mental disorder as follows:

> A mental disorder is a syndrome characterized by clinically significant disturbance in an individual's cognition, emotion regulation, or behavior that reflects a dysfunction in the psychological, biological, or developmental processes underlying mental functioning. Mental disorders are usually associated with significant distress or disability in social, occupational, or other important activities. An expectable or culturally approved response to a common stressor or loss, such as the death of a loved one, is not a mental disorder. Socially deviant behavior (e.g., political, religious, or sexual) and conflicts that are primarily between the individual and society are not mental disorders unless the deviance or conflict results from a dysfunction in the individual. (Kilgus & Rea, 2014, p. 6)

The definition has been developed considerably since the previous editions of the system, partly in an attempt to meet Wakefield's critique as spelled out in the previous chapter, and the definition now includes reference to "dysfunction". But the problem remains that what one "has", when suffering from a mental disorder, is solely identified with symptoms – or even (at least as long as no clear biomarkers have been identified) *is* these symptoms. Concerning somatic illness there is a reasonably firm difference between symptoms and illness: pain and difficulties walking can be symptoms of a bone fracture in the leg (but also of many other things); fatigue and night sweats may be symptoms of cancer (but also of many other things). It is common to talk about "symptomatic treatment" as inadequate, since it does not really target the illness itself that lies behind the symptoms and creates them. In psychiatry, however, there is by and large an identity between symptoms and illness. Inattentiveness, hyperactivity and lack of impulse control are not only symptoms of ADHD; they *are* ADHD, if they are severe enough. This means that ADHD as an epistemic object, like other psychiatric conditions, is constituted by symptoms: if one has the symptoms, then one has the disorder, and vice versa.

The next aspect concerns identity. I shall return to "psychiatric identity" in Chapter 5, so for now I will simply try to make the point that one may not only *have* ADHD, but also that one may *be* ADHD, or at least hyperactive, impulsive etc. In Danish it is common to say: "I am an ADHDer" in the same way that one may say: "I am a footballer". When I began to conduct fieldwork in a support group for adults diagnosed with ADHD,[1] it was immediately obvious how many group members self-identified and identified each other using the diagnostic category (much more about this in Chapter 4), but although an "ADHD identity" is common in this group, it is important to add that I do not believe that one could say that their subjectivity in total (whatever that could signify) is determined through the ADHD diagnosis. Obviously, many other categories are also important in framing people's identities (such as mother, father, student, unemployed, divorced etc.), but the diagnosis does enter into people's self-understanding as one significant component.

Finally, there is the action aspect, related to the idea that people do not just have mental disorders, or identify with them, but they are also something people *do* or *perform* relative to certain norms related to specific categories such as ADHD, depression or personality disorders. This aspect can easily be misunderstood, since we – or the diagnosed – do not in general experience sufferings as something we *do*. However, researchers such as Emily Martin, herself diagnosed with bipolar disorder

---

1   Since 2013, I have conducted fieldwork in a support group for adults diagnosed with ADHD in Denmark. The group meets every month, and, in addition to participating in regular group meetings, I have also recruited a number of key informants through the support group that I have interviewed in greater depth about living with the ADHD diagnosis. In Chapters 4 and 7 of this book in particular, I unfold some of the findings based on the fieldwork.

and who has written a fascinating account of this diagnosis in American society, emphasize the performative aspect as particularly important. Martin explains how her informants "were able to perform mania in a situationally appropriate way, commenting through meta-action on the condition itself" (Martin, 2007, p. 86). Her informants, for example in self-help groups, were neither helpless victims of the disorder "nor so medicated that they were incapable of displaying mania" (p. 86); rather, they could calibrate their mania to the ways that were deemed appropriate in the local moral worlds of self-help groups, although sometimes they would "break the rules" and be corrected. It is very interesting how a diagnosis on the one hand may take responsibility away from people (because they are seen as manic, for example), but on the other hand embodies norms that dictate which behaviours are appropriate and which are not for a specific kind of suffering. This presupposes a large degree of responsibility understood as capabilities for action and reflexive self-consciousness.

In a Danish study of psychiatric institutions, Agnes Ringer (2013) has shown how the patients learn to perform their conditions in a way that is perceived as adequate in the eyes of the professionals, precisely in order to be able to receive treatments. If they act in a way that is seen as "too well", they risk being discharged against their will, but if they act in a way that is "too ill", they risk being seen as fakers that simply exaggerate their symptoms. It is probably quite general for psychiatric diagnoses that people diagnosed must learn to act properly as mentally disordered in situationally required ways – relative to the concrete social practices in which one participates (family, work, contact with social workers, self-help groups, clinics etc.). One must learn how to perform one's suffering properly, and the diagnosis provides a significant "script" in this regard. I do not put it this way to imply that people diagnosed do not suffer – sadly, they surely do – but rather to emphasize that forms of suffering that may be idiosyncratic or diffuse become aligned with authoritative models such as those made explicit in the diagnostic manuals, and this is institutionalized in self-help groups, in psychoeducative projects (see Jensen, 2015) and many other places in our diagnostic cultures.

The idea of articulating these three aspects is to emphasize both that mental disorder and human suffering in general may encompass all three, and that a single one of these aspects will often become salient within certain specific social practices. For example, participating in the work of patient organizations (such as self-help or support groups) can often lead to the identity aspect becoming prevalent. One normally gains access to such a group because one identifies with it, and the dynamics in the group can help establish that "here we are ADHD people together" (Brinkmann, 2014b). In other contexts of life (for example, on the football field), the ADHD diagnosis might simply not be very relevant and is not brought into play, while people diagnosed will sometimes even distance themselves from it. In my fieldwork among adults diagnosed with ADHD, I have found that people employ the diagnosis very flexibly and switch between mobilizing the three aspects of the disorder to which the diagnosis is open: in some contexts, they *have* ADHD, in others they *are* "ADHD people" and sometimes they are conscious of the ways that ADHD should be *done* properly (both in relation to others so diagnosed and in relation to the system of treatment; see Chapter 4 for examples).

It is important to be aware how focusing on just a single aspect at the expense of the others can lead to different risks for the diagnosed. If mental disorders are just something people *have*, the risk is a problematic entification; that is, treating the problem or suffering as a "thing" one "has". However, if no such concrete "thing" can be identified scientifically, which very often is the case in psychiatry (besides purely behavioural symptoms), the diagnosed people risk being approached as whiners or fakers who simply wish to "exploit the system" or something similar. (This is a particular problem in relation to so-called functional or somatoform disorders, where patients experience bodily symptoms but without any "objective" way to corroborate them.) With psychiatric disorders such as ADHD, the diagnosis is formulated on the basis of symptoms, where different tests are used as tools, but it is unclear (for the diagnosed but also for professionals and researchers) whether ADHD refers to anything beyond the set of symptoms. Nevertheless (as we shall also see later in this book), the diagnosis (here, ADHD as a category) is often used to explain the symptoms experienced by the patients, which, however, is completely circular and thus empty. The reason is that the diagnosis is formulated on the basis of symptoms, and is thus not able to explain the same set of symptoms (Timimi, 2009). The symptoms are *signs* of illness or disorder and diagnoses are *names* for illness or disorder, and there may arise a circular relationship between signs and names, whereby they mutually refer to each other. Not only people diagnosed (as we shall see later), but also representatives of the system of treatment at large report that the ADHD diagnosis provides an "explanation" for problems that might always have existed in a person's life, but, strictly speaking, this is not the case, because of the descriptive rather than explanatory nature of diagnoses. Diagnoses simply redescribe symptoms using the different psychiatric categories.

A unique and exclusive focus on the identity aspect – seeing a mental disorder as something one simply *is* – can lead to a risk of chronification. It may become quite difficult to relate to oneself as something besides mentally disordered, if one's identity is constituted around a diagnostic category. How can one then develop *from* the diagnosis? The Norwegian psychologist Arnhild Lauveng writes in her book *Tomorrow I Was Always a Lion* about her life as a schizophrenic, and she begins by stating that the reason for writing the book is that she is a *former* schizophrenic, which sounds almost as impossible as "former AIDS patient" – it is something that hardly exists (Lauveng, 2008). When she was ill, it was an established "truth" in the psychiatric system that schizophrenic was something one *was* (identity) and that it was chronic. Although the symptoms of schizophrenia may last for years, there is hardly any doubt that it may itself contribute to fixating an "illness identity" if the story of chronicity is the only one the patient is told by authorities in the system of treatment. Fortunately, much has happened since, but for many disorders (among them ADHD and autism spectrum disorders), there is more or less scientific consensus that the condition is innate and chronic. This may be correct (or not), but in any case the point is that it may make other identity options impossible if the diagnostic identity comes to be dominant.

If the risk of chronification and "patient identity" arises when the identity aspect becomes dominant, it is more or less the reverse problem that follows from a unique focus on the performative aspect. For if mental illness is "just" something people *do*, then it seems that they are free to do something else, or do what they do in a different, non-pathological, way. This is a common reaction to the performative aspect and one of the reasons why those social constructionists, who put all weight on this aspect, are often accused of neglecting the fact that patients can in fact be locked in patterns that they do not control and that they just cannot reconstruct. There is a risk that one downplays human suffering if only the performative aspect is recognized, and this may lead to an overburdening of the patient with responsibility for coping and recovery.

Do Psychiatric Diagnoses Refer to Natural Kinds?

I shall now move on from the three dimensions of diagnoses to address the question about the status of diagnoses as epistemic objects. Do they refer to what philosophers call "natural kinds" or are they something else? This question can be addressed by taking a look at Ian Hacking's work on the theme. (What follows is based on Brinkmann, 2005.) Asking whether diagnoses pick out natural kinds represents another way of asking whether the idea of disease specificity (discussed by Rosenberg) applies to psychiatric disorders. If so, they can be said to be natural kinds.

But what are natural kinds? Paradigm examples include such things as tigers, water or gold. They are "groups of naturally occurring phenomena that inherently resemble each other and differ crucially from other phenomena" (Danziger, 1999, p. 80). It is one of the goals of natural science to discover and identify natural kinds, and it is a distinctive mark of the natural sciences *that* they are able to identify these. As Karl Marx famously said: "All science would be superfluous if the outward appearance and the essence of things directly coincided" (Marx, 1971, p. 817). The search for natural kinds is the search for the underlying essences of things. We (as knowledge-seeking humans) want to find natural kinds, because, if we succeed in doing so, we have an overview of the common essential properties of a class of things (for example, an underlying disease) that allow us to explain other, more superficial, properties of this class of things (for example, psychiatric symptoms). Take water as an example. Water has certain observable properties: it is colourless, tasteless, has a specific boiling point and freezing point and so on. The underlying essential property that allows us to explain all these "superficial" properties is its molecular structure (H_2O). Scientific categories can be said to refer to natural kinds if it is conceivable that we could discover that what these terms refer to, in fact have completely different properties from what we have traditionally thought, without this making us use a different term to name them

(Collin, 1990). For example, if humans developed finer senses of taste, and found that water is not really tasteless, we would still call it water. The reason for this is that its underlying essence remains the same, although its "superficial" phenomenal properties appear differently.

The discussion of natural kinds has been significant in modern linguistic philosophy, challenging widespread views of linguistic meaning. Most philosophers (and also cognitive psychologists) have thought that meanings are mental entities of some sort. Knowing the meaning of "water" would, on this traditional account, involve being in a certain psychological state, or having a certain mental representation. The philosophers Saul Kripke and Hilary Putnam successfully challenged this view in the early 1970s. Putnam, on whom I concentrate here, asserted: "Cut the pie any way you like, 'meanings' just ain't in the head!" (Putnam, 1973, p. 704). Putnam defended an externalist account of meaning on the grounds that the meaning of such terms as "water" could not be accounted for as concepts, or indeed mental entities of any kind. Instead their meanings had to be understood as rigidly fixed to the natural kind picked out by the term. The illustrative and now-famous science-fiction example given by Putnam is the "Twin-Earth" example. He asks us to imagine that an expedition from our planet Earth finds another planet far away from ours, which in every detail is just like our planet. They name it Twin-Earth. On that planet, there is a liquid, which in all immediate phenomenal respects is just like our water. People on Twin-Earth have exactly the same practices with this liquid as we have with water on our planet. They drink it, boil it and freeze it, just like we do. But when the expedition analyses the liquid chemically, it turns out that its molecular structure is not H_2O, but XYZ. The question, then, is: how should the compound be classified? Putnam argued that we would intuitively say, and rightly so, that the compound is not water, but merely something that looks just like it in all observable respects. Putnam thus argued that natural kind terms (such as "water") refer to natural kinds ("essences", such as "H_2O"), just as proper names refer to particular people, without the mediation of mentally represented meanings or definitions (Haslam, 1998). These terms are rigidly fixed to their referents.

If we accept this analysis of natural kind terms, the next question to ask is whether diagnostic terms, or other terms used in psychology and psychiatry, refer to natural kinds – and here the answer seems to be no (Collin, 1990). As things stand, we have little reason to believe that any of the terms used in the human and social sciences, including psychiatry, refer to natural kinds. Why so? Let me explain by invoking an example. It would not be conceivable to think that we could discover that a *hospital* is really not an institution whose purpose it is to treat illnesses, but something completely different, say, a place for developing means for biological warfare. If it turns out that some hospital *de facto* functions like this, we will have to conclude, not that we did not know what hospitals were, but that this specific institution was not a hospital. Even a Foucauldian unmasking of the rise of treatment institutions in modernity cannot make things otherwise. If some radical Foucauldian could show that all hospitals in fact have worked single-mindedly to oppress rather than cure people, the right conclusion would be that *bona fide* hospitals have never existed, only institutions calling themselves "hospitals"', but with different, "un-hospital-like" underlying rationales.

To take an example closer to our diagnostic cultures theme: it seems unlikely that we would say, even if we one day succeeded in identifying depression with a specific neural dysfunction, that we had thereby discovered a natural kind (the essence of depression). This is because, to reiterate the Twin-Earth example, if it turns out that depressed people on Twin-Earth, people with anhedonia and all other phenomenal expressions of depression, have a completely different neuronal make-up from depressed people on Earth, then we would still not give up our classification of these people as depressed. They would still be rightly described as "depressed" even though their neuronal structure corresponded to the neuronal structure of happy and carefree people on Earth. Unlike water, there is not in the case of depression a natural kind, some underlying essence, which fixes the meaning of the concept "depression". Instead, its meaning is tied to the "superficial", observable properties of depressed behaviour and its significance in the human life world. In this regard, it is impossible to separate the "superficial" phenomenal properties and some underlying "essential" properties when it comes to diagnoses and other human concepts. This seems to be their fate as epistemic objects. The problem is, so to speak, that the mental problems of human beings are identified with, and constituted by, their "symptoms", as these are phenomenally visible, and not by anything behind these. In the psy-sciences, concepts cannot be about some completely hidden essence, because, as Anthony Giddens has argued about concepts in the social sciences across the board, they are *concepts about concepts* (Giddens, 1976). That is, they are concepts that somehow *must* hook up with the participants' own concepts. (This argument was also forcefully made by Peter Winch, 1963.) Understanding the phenomena addressed in psychology, psychiatry, and the social sciences always means understanding *from within* the practices and cultures researched.

Diagnostic categories thus have to relate to the phenomena of the life world and with "folk psychologies", but if psychiatric and psychological categories do not refer to hidden essences or natural kinds, then what do they refer to? Famously, Hacking has answered that they refer to human kinds. (He has since changed his terminology and now talks about "interactive kinds", but I shall here stick to his original formulation.) What are these? Initially, we can outline three ways in which human kinds differ from natural kinds:

Natural kinds:
- Intelligible outside discursive contexts
- Indifferent to the descriptions applied to them
- Categories and kinds are independent

Human kinds:
- Intelligible only within a discursive context

- Interact with the descriptions applied to them
- Categories and kinds emerge together

Hacking says that "the chief difference between natural and human kinds is that the human kinds often make sense only within a certain social context" (Hacking, 1995b, p. 362). One can be a captain or a samurai, for example, only in certain social settings, where certain discourses and descriptions are available. One can be a king only in a world where the institution of monarchy exists (water, on the other hand, was H_2O before the institution of chemistry). Human kinds indicate "kinds of people, their behaviour, their condition, kinds of action, kinds of temperament or tendency, kinds of emotion, and kinds of experience" (pp. 351–352). As mentioned above, Hacking has analyzed in varying detail "multiple personality disorder" (Hacking, 1995a), "fugue" (Hacking, 1998), "homosexuality" (Hacking, 1986), "suicide", "teen-age pregnancy", "adolescence", "child abuse", "autism" and "Hispanic" (Hacking, 1995b) as concrete examples of human kinds.

An important feature of human kinds is that they can exert effects on themselves (Martin & Sugarman, 2001). They are affected by their classifications and interact with their classifications, sometimes affecting the classifications themselves. Human kinds can even intentionally try to change how they are classified (for instance, when homosexuals objected to being categorized as pathological through diagnoses). This is the looping effect of human kinds: "People classified in a certain way tend to conform to or grow into the ways they are described; but they also evolve in their own ways, so that the classifications and descriptions have to be constantly revised" (Hacking, 1995a, p. 21). And further: "Inventing or molding a new kind, a new classification, of people or of behavior may create new ways to be a person, new choices to make, for good or evil. There are new descriptions, and hence new actions under a description" (p. 239).

Why do new kinds of description, for example, those produced by psychiatrists and psychologists – Hacking (1995b) refers to Freud as "the king of the loopers" – provide for new kinds of action? Because in so far as human actions are *intentional*, they are *actions under a description* (Hacking, 1995a, p. 234). We only say that people act intentionally if they are able to provide some kind of description of their action that renders it meaningful by locating it in a discursive context. I can only have the intention to vote for a given candidate at a democratic election if I can describe the physical behaviour commonly associated with voting (going to the voting booth and marking the piece of paper) as an act of voting. One cannot act intentionally under a description unless this description is discursively available. As Hacking says:

> When new descriptions become available, when they come into circulation, or even when they become the sorts of things that it is all right to say, to think, then there are new things to choose to do. When new intentions become open to me, because new descriptions, new concepts, become available to me, I live in a world of new opportunities. (Hacking, 1995a, p. 236)

Hacking is clear that this does not amount to any facile social constructionism, and this is where he – as I aim to do in this book – tries to steer a course between essentialism and constructionism. He characterizes himself as a realist (Hacking, 1986). Human kinds are indeed very real, and although we are in the business of potentially making up new kinds of people when we invent new classifications and new "fields of description" (Hacking, 1995b), this does not make the kinds any less real. Some people have in fact suffered from Multiple Personality Disorder, which is the condition he has described and analyzed in the greatest detail. They (and the communities in which they live) were not faking it, although they could not have acted the way they did, and *eo ipso* suffered from this condition, before the relevant "field of description" became available sometime late in the 19th century – or to be precise, late in the afternoon of July 27, 1885, when Charcot's student, Jules Voisin, described the very first MPD-patient, Louis Vivet (Hacking, 1995a, p. 171). In contrast, it can reasonably be argued that people were able to suffer from tuberculosis even before this illness was named (although they may have been unaware of the cause of their disease). In the case of tuberculosis there is a relevant natural kind involved that causes the disease, which is not dependent on a discursive context; that is to say, on how it is described and classified. In other words, in the case of tuberculosis, there is a distinction to be made between disease and symptoms, whereas this is not similarly the case with regard to psychiatric problems.

Nonetheless, it is important to bear in mind that human kinds, for Hacking, are just as real as natural kinds. There is no ontological difference between them in that sense. Human kinds do not belong to a different, "non-natural" world. In a sense they are just as natural as natural kinds, but they are natural in a different way, perhaps akin to what Hegel and modern Hegelians call "second nature" (Hegel, 1821, p. 35; McDowell, 1994); that is, nature as it expresses itself in and through social practices (through processes of semiotic mediation, for example, as I emphasize in this book). Human kinds as second nature entities are no less natural than natural kinds (first nature entities), nor are they necessarily easier to change. If our category "white rhinoceros" refers to a natural kind, then we can wipe out all instances of this natural kind quite easily – unfortunately all too easily. Sadly, we cannot similarly eliminate depression, although "depression" is a human kind term. Moreover, the fact that depression is not a natural kind does not make the condition any less serious for those who suffer from it. The distinction between natural and human kinds tells us absolutely nothing about either the ontological "persistency" of any of these kinds, or the "seriousness" of their existence.

I should add that not everyone agrees that psychiatric diagnoses are incapable of picking out natural kinds. The collection of papers edited by Harold Kincaid and Jacqueline Sullivan presents many different perspective on exactly this discussion, but based on the argument outlined above, I agree with those like Haslam, who argues that it is highly unlikely that we can discover natural kinds in psychiatry for both conceptual and empirical reasons (Haslam, 2014). Haslam makes an interesting observation that gives an additional pragmatic reason to be suspicious of the natural kind talk in psychiatry: based on a number of studies of lay persons' attitudes to mental disorders, he argues not only that the folk psychiatric idea of mental disorder is a variant of an essentialist natural kind theory (people tend to believe that mental disorders are discrete diseases within people, cf. the notion of disease specificity), but also that this idea is deeply harmful because it increases stigmatization. Intuitively, one could think the opposite – that conceiving of mental disorders as "illnesses like any other" would reduce stigma by reducing moral blame and increasing sympathy – but it turns out that an essentialist, natural kind idea of mental disorder instead encourages stigma because, Haslam says, "it represents sufferers as categorically abnormal, immutably afflicted, and essentially different" (p. 25). If this is true (and many studies have now been conducted that back this conclusion) it gives us an additional pragmatic and even ethical reason not to take for granted that psychiatric diagnoses refer to natural kinds.

Creating Disorders as Human Kinds

If psychiatric diagnoses refer to human kinds as their epistemic objects, how, then, do these come into the world? This will be the final question of this chapter.

The three aspects that I have highlighted above (having, being, doing) concern both diagnoses and disorders (or illnesses): they are aspects of the experience of being *diagnosed* and thereby involve a psychiatric category, but they are also aspects of what it means to *suffer* from the disorders or illnesses. And, as I have tried to demonstrate with the discussion of human kinds and their looping effects, the relationship between diagnoses and disorders is extremely complex and dynamic. I shall now approach this relationship head-on by focusing on those processes that enable something to emerge as a psychiatric disorder, not in the lives of the afflicted (this is studied, for example, in the discipline of developmental psychopathology), but in the cultural systems of social practices which have historically been developed to handle people's problems.

In one of the few thorough discussions of the sociology of diagnoses, Annemarie Jutel has described the role of diagnoses in modern society (Jutel, 2011). One of the functions of diagnoses – both for professionals and the diagnosed themselves – is to transform clusters of perhaps coincidental symptoms into an organized illness. This is probably what is implied when people consistently say that a diagnosis provides an explanation of the suffering, because it seems that people understand their problems better when they somehow get "assembled" through the diagnostic category. However, saying that the diagnosis "assembles" the symptoms suggests that it operates actively in the lives of the diagnosed and does not just describe a pre-existing reality neutrally. To use Parsons' classical term, the diagnosis provides access to a sick role, and in this way allows one to be ill, and it may also contribute to rearranging the individual's identity (p. 11). Gaining access to the sick role can involve both a process of biographical disruption, but also one of narrative reconstruction through the scripts offered by the diagnostic terms (Jutel & Nettleton, 2011, p. 794).

Jutel emphasizes three conditions that must be in place on a societal scale in order for something to become a disorder that can be characterized diagnostically (Jutel, 2011, p. 35): (1) First, there must be a common recognition that the condition is undesirable. In most cases, something is deemed undesirable, because it creates suffering or impairs normal functioning for the person herself, but it can also be the case that the condition creates a problem for others. This might be so for personality disorders, for example anti-social personality disorder, but it can also be the case when children are diagnosed (for example, with ADHD), where it is often not the children themselves who experience anything particularly negative that calls for a diagnosis. With this first condition, we are close to Wakefield's first component as discussed above (that is, that something is harmful).

(2) Second, there must be a technical capacity to discern the condition. In other words, tools and technologies are necessary to make the condition visible, which was also underlined in Danziger's analysis of epistemic objects. It is no use having an illness category if there is no way to identify and recognize the problem across cases. In psychiatry, with its lack of reliable biomarkers, the dominating technology is today the symptom checklist. Many different tests have been developed as tools to formulate a psychiatric diagnosis, which often happens together with a thorough examination based on anamnesis. In recent decades, however, standardized tests have come to play a larger and larger role at the expense of the doctor's clinical judgment. (In Chapter 5, I look more closely at what happens when persons begin to understand themselves in light of the quantitative measures used to assess their symptoms.) But it is not just in psychiatry that the technical capacity is important. Jutel mentions scales as a precondition of being overweight coming to constitute a medically relevant condition. Human beings have always varied concerning their bodies, but with scales becoming common as a means to measure people's weight and the invention of the body mass index (BMI), the technology exists to make obesity into a medical category. The history of the BMI is interesting in itself, and it represents a general development whereby diagnostic criteria are expanded to include more and more people. Although studies indicate that mortality is actually lower for (moderately) overweight people (BMI 30–34.9) than for people with so-called "normal" weight, the upper limit of "healthy" weight has changed from 27.8 kg/m2 in 1990 to 24.9 kg/m2 (Jutel, 2011, p. 46).

The technical capacity to discern something as an illness sometimes consists of the very availability of a way of treating the condition. For example, there is a widespread belief about ADHD that the "proof" that someone really suffers from this disorder is that the medicine for treating the symptoms (notably methylphenidate) actually works and enables the person to concentrate better and control his or her impulses, when compared to the effects of the medicine on people who do not have the diagnosis. Much, however, indicates that this is a myth, and that the medicine has more or less the same effects on everyone (which also explains why there is a market for the medicine as a "cognitive enhancer" in relation to exams, for example). The sociologist Peter Conrad, who has analyzed the medicalization of society, writes about how the medical industry has often developed products to target specific conditions before these conditions are classified as illnesses or disorders. Conrad predicts that we will see a growth of the diagnosis "Memory deficit disorder" once scientists develop a drug to enhance memory pharmacologically (Conrad, 2007, p. 72). He quotes Gerald Yakatan (CEO of the pharmaceutical company Avanir) who states explicitly about ADHD and other conditions: "Before there were drugs, these conditions didn't exist" (p. 143). Often it is the medical optimization technology in itself that changes our perception of a certain level of functioning into one that sees it as pathological.

(3) The third sociological condition mentioned by Jutel that must be in place in order for something to become a disorder is that there must be a collective will to assimilate it into the ranks of diseases rather than the moral or religious spheres, for example (Jutel, 2011, p. 35). In the next chapter, we shall see that many "languages of suffering" exist with different potentials to render human suffering meaningful, and it seems fair to conclude that we have moved from a situation in which many such languages were available to conceptualize and cope with the problems of life, to one where the diagnostic language has become extremely prevalent and in some cases even hegemonic, coming close to relegating other ways of describing suffering to the periphery. Again, it is obvious to mention ADHD: not long ago unruly children were seen as "naughty boys" (whether this was reasonable or not), whereas now we say that they suffer from ADHD (Timimi, 2009). A moral language has been replaced with a psychiatric language. (Note that I do not here assess whether this is a positive or negative development; I only notice that it has occurred).

In general, the analysis in this chapter is neutral concerning the question of whether it is legitimate to transform a condition into a disorder through a diagnostic category. The point is simply to emphasize that a condition (very rarely) in itself communicates that it is a psychiatric disorder. Concerning many psychiatric disorders, in particular those such as ADHD that have been growing in recent years, researchers tend to disagree. Some believe that the disorder has always been there, but that we (doctors and other psy-professionals) have only discovered it recently. Others believe that the condition may always have been there, but never as a disorder as such, so that what has happened is a medicalization and pathologization of a common human phenomenon rather than identification of an illness. When Jutel argues the sociological point that something does not become a psychiatric disorder unless there are (1) suffering persons involved, (2) a technical capacity to discern it as a disorder, and (3) a collective will to classify it as a disorder, classifying something as a disorder in a normative sense can concretely be seen as fair or unfair. Perhaps it is fair to tell the story of how schizophrenia was constituted as a disorder without wishing to question this development in itself (many will see this as progress compared to older theories of moral depravation and devil worshipping), whereas it can hardly be fair to tell the story of how homosexuality was constituted as a mental disorder on the basis of the three factors mentioned here without critically questioning this line of development (which ended in the 20th century, when homosexuality was gradually removed from the diagnostic manuals).

We can now return to Hacking's different studies of the rise of various psychiatric disorders such as multiple personality disorder (Hacking, 1995a) and fugue (Hacking, 1998), the latter being what he calls a transient mental illness that emerged in the 19th century, spread, and then disappeared again in around 25 years (the symptoms having included travelling from one place to another, often long distances, without being able to restrain oneself). Hacking shows in his analyses how new ways of being human emerge together with new forms of description (not least diagnoses) and accompanying social practices in which these forms of description make sense. For Hacking there is a looping effect between classification and classified, at least when we talk about responsive human beings (and not, say, molecules that are also classified by chemists), which means that humans can react to being classified (and, for example, either align themselves with the classification or distance themselves from it), which can lead to a need for new classifications, when the old ones no longer match the reality they were meant to describe (Hacking, 1995b).

Hacking analyzes the rise of mental disorders as related to social or ecological "niches" within which a person (in my terminology) can *have*, *be* and *do* mental disorder (Hacking, 1998, p. 13). Mental disorder thus has what Hacking calls "historical ontology" and appears in a niche that is at the same time social, medical, and personal and which offers a stable "home" for certain types of illness manifestation (p. 13). These niches are in other words socio-material practices within which Jutel's three conditions can become manifest and enable something to appear as a mental disorder. The central thesis of this book can now be explicated more specifically: we witness the creation of ecological niches in ever more corners of society, that invite us to see forms of distress and eccentricity as psychiatric problems that can be diagnosed. This, in short, is what is meant by the term "diagnostic cultures".

Conclusions

In this chapter I have approached psychiatric diagnoses as epistemic objects – that is, objects of knowledge – by arguing that the current notion of disease specificity is a quite recent invention in the history of medicine. While it might reasonably apply in many corners of somatic medicine, it is generally spurious in psychiatry. The main reason is that psychiatric diagnoses do not (at least in the large majority of cases) refer to natural kinds, which can be demonstrated from the fact that the categories are tied to "superficial" symptoms rather than "underlying" disease mechanisms. In addition, no biomarkers have been found that clearly and reliably link superficial symptoms (subject to cultural and historical interpretations) with underlying objective pathology. This does not mean that the biological, physiological and neurological aspects of mental disorder are unimportant – far from it – but it does make the link between problem (pathology) and category (diagnosis) more complex.

It thus becomes relevant to discuss the sociological conditions that must be in place in order for some problem to appear as a psychiatric disorder, and, following Jutel, I articulated three of these: there must be a recognition of the undesirability of some condition; there must be a technical capacity to discern it; and there must be a collective (for example, professional or institutional) will to assimilate it to the range of diseases or disorders. Hacking's idea of looping effects can be used to depict some of the interactions between people diagnosed, the categories applied to them, and the sociological conditions and ecological niches in which they live their lives. Looping effects do not occur in a uniquely bilateral manner between diagnosed individuals and scientifically developed classifications (diagnoses), for, in Hacking's scheme, experts, knowledge, and institutions are also relevant since they form a web in which ways of being human (and ways of being distressed) are made and moulded (to use some of Hacking's favourite terms). Within such webs of suffering persons, institutions, professionals and modern welfare states, ways of having, being and doing mental disorders appear. The next chapter looks more directly at some of the clusters of discourses (vocabularies or "languages") and practices that human beings employ to articulate and make sense of their suffering and distress.

Chapter 3
Languages of Suffering

In a discussion of psychiatric "disorders without borders", Nikolas Rose argues that:

> At any time and place, human discontents are inescapably shaped, moulded, given expression, judged and responded to in terms of certain languages of description and explanation, articulated by experts and authorities, leading to specific styles and forms of intervention. What, then, is specific to today? (Rose, 2006, p. 479)

By invoking the notion of "languages of description and explanation" that shape human discontents, Rose hints at what I shall here address as "languages of suffering"; that is to say, vocabularies that we use to interpret, make sense of, and regulate our experiences of distress, discontents or what Thomas Szasz famously called "problems in living" (Szasz, 1961). Rose's own recent work has pointed to the roles of biomedicine (Rose, 2007) and the neurosciences (Rose & Abi-Rached, 2013) in shaping our current ideas of mental disorder and also our very image of what a human being is. According to Rose, the human being is becoming a "neurochemical self" (Rose, 2003). Peter Conrad's influential analysis of the medicalization of society (Conrad, 2007) is now being developed into analyses of biomedicalization and pharmaceuticalization (Abraham, 2010), emphasizing the functions of *Big Pharma* in defining health and illness for people in the 21st century.

Another significant voice, offering critical comment on these developments from inside psychiatry, is David Healy's, whose recent book, *Pharmageddon* not only critically discusses the pharmaceutical industry and the emerging hegemony of evidence-based medicine (to which I return in Chapter 6), but also delivers something like a cultural critique of the ways that the human experience of suffering is now changing in societies that increasingly draw upon biomedical resources when seeking to understand somatic and mental health:

> In previous times we passed on a culture to our children embodied in fairy tales, folklore about health, national myths, and religious precepts, in which the life's risks were put in a larger context of meaning. Now an increasing part of what is transmitted centers on personal health for its own sake: figures for sugar and lipid levels, as increasing numbers of our children have diabetes or other dangerous metabolic states, or figures for peak respiratory flows as increasing numbers of young people have asthma, or statistics on some chemical imbalance as increasing numbers are being treated for ADHD, depression, or anxiety. Not

only is such a culture two-dimensional, it changes the very nature of human experience. (Healy, 2012, p. 176)

According to Healy, the processes of biomedicalization and pharmaceuticalization are reducing the multi-dimensional phenomena of life to a two-dimensional one. Today, "personal troubles" (to borrow a term from Mills, 1959) are routinely pathologized, and behaviours that are seen as disturbing in the eyes of the majority are transformed into mental disorders (Busfield, 2011, p. 5). Critics, such as those cited here, explicitly or implicitly argue that we are increasingly blinding ourselves to dimensions of human distress that cannot be conceived within a psychiatric and diagnostic framework. But it is rarely discussed what these other dimensions are. Through which languages can they be articulated? And what would we gain – if anything – by retrieving some of the other (non-psychiatric) languages of suffering? These are some of the questions that I set out to address in this chapter that aims to map a number of different languages of suffering.

By drawing on the pragmatist and hermeneutic dimensions of cultural psychology, I will first explain in greater detail what I mean by a "language of suffering". Then, I will give a more precise characterization of the common psychiatric understanding of suffering, concentrating here on what I call the "diagnostic language" of psychiatry, which has become very influential in defining human distress. I will emphasize at the outset that my point is *not* to say that this language is useless or illegitimate, but rather that it is simply one among a large range of languages that are valuable in enabling us to understand various dimensions of human life and its problems. The following sections present and unfold some of these other languages, including religious, existential, moral and political languages. Obviously, the list of languages of suffering addressed here is not exhaustive, and the categories are not monolithic or defined by strict boundaries. Still, I hope that it is clear that they represent different aspects of human life and suffering that are important to bear in mind when seeking to fully understand the problems that people face. I end by discussing what roles the different languages ought to play in both theoretical and practical contexts in relation to human distress.

Although the chapter develops and operates with a notion of "languages" that is close to the notion of "discourses" found in different varieties of discourse analysis, I should make clear now that unlike discourse studies as such, this chapter is not based on readings of empirical materials. Doing so has obvious strengths, and many interesting studies of psychiatric discourses have appeared based on discourse analysis, but I believe that my approach to more overarching vocabularies and hermeneutic frameworks in the present chapter is also legitimate and inscribes itself as part of a social psychological and sociological tradition of discussing and theorizing the relationship between society and culture on the one hand and categories of social pathologies (Keohane & Petersen, 2013) and diagnoses (Jutel, 2011) on the other. I return to this issue in the next section, where I discuss the very concept of languages of suffering.

What is a Language of Suffering?

Obviously, I am not the first to suggest that it is fruitful to develop a notion of languages of suffering. In cultural psychology, Richard Shweder and co-workers have for years worked to articulate and refine a distinction between what they refer to as the "Big three" cultural metanarratives of suffering (Shweder, 2008; Shweder, Much, Mahapatra & Park, 1997). The "Big three" are traditions that explain suffering across the divide between somatic and mental health problems, and they highlight the immense variety concerning how (what we call) mental illness and suffering are conceptualized. According to Shweder, the three main metanarratives are: (1) The biomedical narrative, according to which suffering is explained as a result of material events (such as harmful molecular processes in the body), (2) the moral narrative, which frames suffering as a consequence of a breach in the moral order (as expressed in the Buddhist idea of karma, for example), and (3) the interpersonal narrative that refers to magic, witchcraft or spirits as driving forces behind experienced suffering (Shweder, Much, Mahapatra & Park, 1997, p. 127). Most people in the imagined hemisphere of the West today subscribe to some version of (1), but Shweder has estimated that only around 15 per cent of the world's explanations of suffering belong in this category. Most conceptualizations of suffering draw upon the moral and interpersonal metanarratives, so the world is still "superstitious" when seen through the prism of Western science. Metanarratives (1) and (3) share the assumption that suffering is *causally* inflicted (either by molecules or magical techniques), whereas (2) distinguishes itself by framing suffering as a *meaningful* (rather than causal) phenomenon, invoking some notion of a cosmic order that can be breached or polluted. (I return to this fundamental distinction below.)

Although the psychiatric understanding of mental problems has become hugely influential, building on a biomedical narrative, it is significant that there used to be much more openness in our culture to the moral understanding in particular, and its associated treatments. Early forms of mental treatment were significantly called *moral treatment*, and were particularly associated with the names of Tuke (England), Pinel (France), and Chiarugi (Italy) in the first half of the 19th century (Lilleleht, 2003). The term "moral" then signified something much broader than our contemporary understanding of morality (as the human and social sciences were seen as belonging to "the moral sciences"), but moral treatment was nonetheless based on explicit moral values, and "involved the creation and administration of corrective experience within a specialized setting" (p. 169). Pioneers of psychiatric treatment practised a kind of moral cure, which involved work and occupational therapy, general encouragement and a gradual moral edification of the patients' characters. In short, people's suffering was framed within a moral rather than a medical discourse. Modern forms of psychotherapy have since evolved in two main directions, both of them departing from the original basis in moral values. The first direction is that of medical health care, where morality became significantly downplayed as moral "sinners" became psychiatric "degenerates" and morality was "medicalized" in the course of the 19th century (Rimke & Hunt, 2002). The second direction is the humanistic one, where psychotherapy became a secular technology of self-realization, incarnated most clearly in Carl Rogers' client-centred therapy (Brinkmann, 2008). This, however, has only played a minor role within psychiatric settings, but has had huge impact on Western culture as a whole.

My emphasis here on *languages* of suffering is inspired by the pragmatist notion of vocabularies, articulated most forcefully by Richard Rorty (1979). For a pragmatist like Rorty, our ways of understanding and acting in the world are mediated by the linguistic resources at our disposal. Vocabularies – like other human inventions – are tools that do not simply copy the world, but which are useful (or not) in enabling us to cope with the world, to use the catch-phrase made famous by Rorty. Within cultural psychology, as we have seen, this process is conceptualized as semiotic mediation: the use of signs and symbols to regulate thoughts, feelings and actions concerning important matters (Valsiner, 2007). Stating that something is existential melancholy, for example, implies one set of understandings and possibilities for action, whereas stating that it is clinical depression implies another set. For Rorty, there is ultimately no rational grounding to, or ways of assessing the relative values of, different vocabularies over and above their instrumental roles; that is, how well they enable human beings to reach their goals (of happiness, growth, democratic living, etc.). From the pragmatist's perspective, the relevant question to ask of a vocabulary is not "Is it true?", but "What kinds of experiences and actions does the vocabulary make possible?" This question should be kept in mind throughout this chapter.

What Rorty did not develop, however, was a more specific analysis of how languages or vocabularies become inscribed into societies, social practices and personal understandings. In order to conduct such an analysis, with specific reference to languages of suffering, we need in my view to supplement the pragmatist interest in the workings of vocabularies with a hermeneutic perspective on how languages mediate, and become sedimented in, personal and cultural self-understandings. (The issue of how pragmatism and hermeneutics may supplement each other is difficult, but the reader may consult Brinkmann, 2011a.) This can be said to be the project of cultural psychology, that of uniting a pragmatist perspective on action and activity with a hermeneutic approach to interpretation and semiosis.

The influential hermeneutic philosopher and social theorist Charles Taylor has distinguished between three levels of social understanding, which we may apply to an understanding of suffering in this case: (1) an 'upper' level of explicit doctrines (about society, the cosmos, or suffering), (2) a 'middle' level of the symbolic (expressed in rituals, works of art, and cultural symbols, for example), and (3) a 'lower' level of the habitus (embodied understanding) (Taylor, 1999, p. 167). These three levels of understanding are more or less ordered along a continuum ranging from the implicit to the explicit. At the upper level, we have for example the explicit metanarratives of suffering that Shweder has studied. These are made explicit in scientific articles, diagnostic manuals, and self-help literature for example. At the middle level, we have all the rituals of suffering related to diagnosis, treatment, healing, and a range of cultural activities performed by self-help groups and much more. Finally, we have the embodied level, where suffering is felt and experienced, and where the experience cannot be divorced from the explicit vocabularies and symbolic acts associated with human distress. Together, the explicit, symbolic, and embodied levels constitute our cultural *practices of suffering*; that is, how we *do* suffering, enact, feel, and perform it, but also how we *experience* it and come to *identify* with it, as emphasized in this book's model of three dimensions of suffering (having, being and doing). I stress this in order to counter an idealistic interpretation of the notion of "languages of suffering", according to which this notion refers to explicit language only. From the cultural psychological perspective taken here, languages of suffering work in persons' lives through social practices, with various associated rituals and symbols, and are inscribed into the human body and its habitus. There is no formula for how this happens, and it may happen quite differently in relation to different kinds of problems, but the important point, as Taylor insists, is that we should learn to rethink the relations between "base" and "superstructure", (explicit) ideas and (implicit) material and institutional factors:

> what we see in human history is ranges of human practices that are both at once, that is, material practices carried out by human beings in space and time, and very often coercively maintained, and at the same time, self-conceptions, modes of understanding. (Taylor, 2004, p. 31)

We cannot separate ideas (of demonic possession, ADHD, or other problems) from the institutional and material bases from which such ideas arise and influence our understandings; both are aspects of social practices, and the linguistic articulations of practices (for example, the languages of suffering) necessarily operate within a complex field of social practices with symbolic and embodied aspects.

When articulating the different languages of suffering below – diagnostic, religious, existential, moral and political – I will thus briefly relate each of these languages to the social practices of which they are a part (with their symbolic and embodied aspects), and I will end the chapter by discussing how the various languages and associated practices present people with quite different positions from which to act (thereby returning to the pragmatist theme of the action possibilities opened up by the various languages).

The Diagnostic Language

As the word testifies, a diagnostic language is one that understands suffering in terms of symptoms as listed in the reigning diagnostic manuals (DSM and ICD). The contemporary manuals are constructed around certain key assumptions about mental illness: that there is a boundary between the normal and the sick, that there are discrete mental illnesses, and that psychiatry's focus should primarily be on the biological aspects of mental illness (Angel, 2012, p. 8). As is well known from different sociological and historical studies (Horwitz, 2002; Kutchins & Kirk, 1997), a revolution took place in psychiatry around 1980 with the creation of DSM-III, which replaced the older etiological understanding of mental illness with a purely diagnostic understanding, based on actual symptoms within a given period of time. Before DSM-III a diagnosis was formulated on the background of the patient's biography and his or her experiences, actions and relationships, and psychiatrists often employed theoretical terminology when describing the patient, typically drawn from psychoanalysis. Unfortunately, this diagnostic practice was quite unreliable, which prompted the shift to the diagnostic approach of DSM-III and beyond. Now, a diagnosis is formulated if the patient has at least x number of symptoms from a given list within y weeks or months (depending on the specific diagnostic category).

The increasing influence of psychiatric diagnoses on human self-understanding is connected to a more general development in medical practices. Armstrong (1995) has charted how medicine has developed historically from Library Medicine (with a focus on the classical learning of the physician) to Bedside Medicine (with physicians addressing the concrete problems of illness) and Hospital Medicine (with the establishment of large hospitals at the end of the 18th century) and today to what Armstrong calls Surveillance Medicine of the 20th century and beyond. The latter kind of medicine functions by targeting everyone through screenings, surveys, a focus on risk factors, and a problematization of the normal. People can now diagnose themselves by taking tests in magazines, self-help literature, or on the internet. Or they are diagnosed when taking part in some of the large-scale epidemiological studies, which seemingly demonstrate that in any one year, more than a third of the European population could be diagnosed with a mental or brain disorder (Wittchen, Jacobi & Rehm, 2011) (and there are similar prevalence numbers for the US and many other countries).

For psychiatry, this whole development has meant that the psychiatric language and its diagnostic categories have become more important for our self-understanding than ever before. Terms that have specific meanings within psychiatry, such as "stress", "anxiety", "depression" and "mania" have become part of people's everyday vocabularies. We use such terms to understand our behaviours, reactions and emotions, and those of others. To mention just one example, a recent large-scale study of 122 Danish public schools demonstrates that teachers believe that, on average, 24.9 per cent of their pupils have problems to such an extent that they could be given a psychiatric diagnosis (Nordahl, Sunnevåg, Aasen & Kostøl, 2010). For the boys in particular, the figure is a striking 30.8 percent. Teachers are probably not special in this regard, but represent a tendency to conceive of problems, deviance and eccentricity in diagnostic terms. We should bear in mind that even if this chapter focuses on languages of suffering, it is not necessarily the suffering of the person who has been given the diagnosis that is significant; it can also be how this person inflicts suffering on others (classmates, parent, teachers), although DSM-5 states that socially deviant behaviour is not a mental disorder unless it results from an individual dysfunction (which, however, is extremely difficult to establish, partly due to the lack of biomarkers for mental disorders).

Numerous critics have addressed the psychiatrization of suffering. They have argued that the extreme prevalence estimates mentioned above represent a huge number of false positives, leading to massive pathologization of normality (Wakefield, 2010). This can happen when these estimates become news stories that trigger something like moral panic among politicians, resulting in new processes of screening and intervention, leading to even more people using the diagnostic language to understand themselves and their afflictions in something approaching a vicious diagnostic cycle on the cultural level. Many traits and behaviours that used to be considered normal human problems (sorrow, melancholia, guilt, shyness, etc.) are therefore now conceptualized as mental disorders that can be diagnosed and treated medically and therapeutically.

Other critics focus on the role of the pharmaceutical industry in marketing illnesses, profiting hugely from pathologizing human problems (Ebeling, 2011), perhaps with something like "pharmageddon" as a result (Healy, 2012). Such pathologization runs the risk of "cultivating vulnerability" in human beings that may become less able to tolerate pain and distress as they are constantly on the lookout for emergent symptoms (Furedi, 2004). As Barsky (1988) argued some years ago, there seems to be a "paradox of health", since more and more people historically experience more and more symptoms and subjective distress at the same time as (and perhaps partly because) more and more treatments become available. When new treatments become available along with new diagnostic categories, new ways of suffering emerge that can be "taken up" by individuals in the dynamic process that Hacking has called "the looping effect of human kinds" (Hacking, 1995b), referring to an interaction between categories that designate human doings and sufferings on the one hand and human beings who may act and interpret their lives in light of these categories on the other (see the previous chapter). This invites everyone to see him or herself as a victim or a patient, although this invitation can be resisted and is even attacked by different organizations such as the Hearing Voices Network, which seeks to de-pathologize voice-hearing.

Despite the criticism, we should certainly not forget to inquire into possible benefits that may arise from using the diagnostic language to conceive of human suffering. There are two broad kinds of benefits. One is connected to the functioning of modern welfare societies in which psychiatric diagnoses are often the immediate key to accessing different forms of benefits, ranging from special education to pensions. In relation to this, there is a debate concerning how to weigh the benefits accrued to individuals against the possible skewing of public health resources in the direction of minor mental health problems at the expense of major psychiatric problems (Williams, 2009). Some will argue that the losers are the traditional psychiatric patients (people suffering from schizophrenia, for example) when so many resources are used to treat minor episodes of depression, anxiety, and stress-related disorders. The other category of conceivable benefits concerns the capacity of diagnostic language to "externalize" people's problems through the diagnostic categories. The idea of externalizing has been developed within narrative therapy to help people appreciate that *they* are not the problem, but that "the problem is the problem", as it is often put (White, 2007). A diagnosis may give people a language that can help frame, objectify and externalize the problem so that the sufferer can regain some sense of personal agency and become able to cope with the difficulties. (I return to this in the next chapter with empirical examples.) However, we know very little about when and how a diagnostic process can lead to externalization and reinvigorated agency, and when it leads in the opposite direction: to the possible formation of patient identity, fixing the person in a sick role. So far, we can only say that sometimes, the use of diagnostic language is itself therapeutic (Wykes & Callard, 2010, p. 301), possibly because of its externalizing potential, but sometimes it seems to cultivate passivity and vulnerability (Wainwright & Calnan, 2002).

In summing up the diagnostic language and its implications for cultural understandings of suffering, we can say that this language has worked very efficiently at the explicit level of understanding (cf. Taylor's three levels described above), most obviously with the diagnostic manuals operating as powerful connecting tissues in and between a large number of social practices, and the diagnoses themselves being central boundary objects within many communities of practice of modern societies (Bowker & Star, 2000). But we also see its impact on the levels of the symbolic and ritual, for example, in the many tests that are ritualistically performed to assess mental health in a variety of settings, and not least at the embodied level, where human beings have appropriated the diagnostic language as a form of self-interpretation of suffering. Perhaps even the physical body itself is affected by the diagnostic language, as hinted at by Margaret Lock's concept of "local biologies", highlighting the ways that our embodied experience, including that of illness and health, is mediated by local categories of knowledge (Lock, 2001). People today, for example, easily interpret their "butterflies in the stomach" as anxiety, their weariness as depression, or their inattentiveness as ADHD, representing a kind of embodied "looping effect" (Hacking, 1995b).

In the following sections, I will briefly address four other languages that offer alternative understandings of human suffering, but which have been somewhat depreciated by the status of the diagnostic language.

The Religious Language

In his song *God* from 1970, John Lennon opens with the famous line that "God is a concept by which we measure our pain". This is so important to Lennon that he repeats it in a quite curious way ("I'll say it again: God is a concept..."). From sociological and cultural psychological perspectives, religion has certainly been ascribed many functions such as "social cement", as opium for the people, as exchange and social control (Turner, 1991), but there is no doubt that the capacity of religion to explain and render pain and suffering meaningful is a major sociocultural function of belief systems as articulated through religious languages. Religions provide a way of seeing oneself within a larger horizon of meaning – an *ontic logos* (Taylor, 1989) – that typically explicates the proper (and forbidden) paths of human beings through their lives. Religions can provide people with the "whys" of their lives (in Nietzschean fashion: "if we possess a why of life, we can put up with almost any how"), and they traditionally tell people that even if their sufferings are painful, they are not intolerable because they are a result of God's will, a temporary stage on a path towards salvation or something similar. According to Max Weber, the problem of suffering is the driving force of all religious evolution (see Wilkinson, 2005, p. 2), and Weber referred to "soteriology" as the ways that humans make sense of their sufferings (Rose, 2007, p. 255), somewhat akin to what I address in this book as languages of suffering.

As we saw earlier with reference to Shweder's analyses, religious languages (which will typically belong in his interpersonal category, where spirits and demons may interfere with human affairs) are still very widespread around the world and are used to make sense of human suffering. Clearly, religious language is made explicit in holy scriptures of different kinds, and has a large range of symbolic and ritualistic practices attached to it that can be used to alleviate human problems (ranging from confessions and exorcism to shamanistic rituals and voodoo ceremonies). For the believer, the religious language of suffering is also made personal and embodied as a form of understanding in one's everyday life, and may involve prayers and other symbolic resources (Zittoun, 2006) that people use to semiotically regulate their thoughts, feelings and actions.

A thorough analysis of the religious language of suffering is obviously beyond the scope of this chapter. Suffice it here to say that this language has not disappeared, just as religion has not disappeared in spite of secularization, but instead has become something of a choice that demands personal reasons to be thought of as legitimate. Furthermore, as summarized by Charles Taylor in his *magnum opus* on secularism: "What was formerly sin is often now seen as sickness" (Taylor, 2007, p. 618). This pathologization of the human condition and its problems, which were originally seen as religious, rests on the one hand, as Taylor observes, on a humanist call for dignity and enlightenment, but may on the other hand end up abasing human dignity. How so? Because we might end up with a two-dimensional understanding of human suffering, and experience more broadly, which Søren Kierkegaard famously referred to as "levelling"; a flattening of qualitative distinctions in human life leading to difficulties in understanding differences between the significant and insignificant. (This discussion is continued and expanded in Chapter 5.) This takes us to another language that in some of its dialects is closely related to the religious, *viz*. the existential.

The Existential Language

An existential language of suffering sees various human problems as inescapable parts of our existence. This language may be coupled with a religious sensibility, as was the case with Kierkegaard, or it may be atheist. In any case, the point is that phenomena such as death-anxiety or despair are regarded not as pathological conditions to be treated medically or therapeutically, but as defining features of human life. The capacity for such emotions and experiences is precisely what makes us human. Famously, Kierkegaard wrote about the *Sickness unto Death* (Kierkegaard, 1849), but the sickness in question was not conceived in medical terms (something to be treated with medicine, therapy or exercise, for example), but in existential terms, having to do with problems arising from reflexive selfhood. The sickness; that is, the feeling of despair, is thus the normal, according to Kierkegaard, and not something that hits a few unlucky souls. Likewise, Kierkegaard's analysis of *The Concept of Anxiety* (Kierkegaard, 1844) does not address a psychiatric phenomenon, but concerns an aspect of human existence which is related to finitude and to our confrontation with our own mortality. In Kierkegaard's eyes, this kind of anxiety has literally nothing as its object, which is why it is, in a sense, the gateway to freedom and authenticity (because nothingness is related to the possibility to act, to bring that which does not yet exist into the world). It is not that humans should be constantly mentally tortured by anxiety, but rather that an understanding of our existential depths demands the potential for feelings of this kind.

Anxiety in the face of death reminds us that life is finite, and that we therefore ought to take it seriously. (Only humans can feel anxiety in this object-less way, while the [other] animals can fear specific objects only.) Perhaps the most significant discussion of the possible pathologization of the existential in recent years concerns grief. Grief was included in the appendix to DSM-5, which, critics argue, represents an obvious example of how the diagnostic language can infiltrate an existential issue (Kofod, 2013). As Kofod recounts, bereaved individuals who experience intense longing, sorrow and emotional pain after the first year of their loss might receive a diagnosis called Adjustment Disorder Related to Bereavement – insofar as these experiences are judged by professionals to be disproportionate – or they may be diagnosed with depression, since the so-called bereavement exclusion has now been eliminated from DSM-5. (In DSM-IV this excluded from a diagnosis of depression people who experienced "depressive symptoms" within two months after the death of a loved one.) Although grief is a very painful phenomenon, it seems to be a good example of a human phenomenon that is at the same time deeply meaningful (it maintains an emotional relationship to the deceased), and something most people would not have removed medically if, for example, a pill existed that could eliminate the feeling of grief. "Grief is love that has become homeless", as it is sometimes put (in Danish, here translated), so the painful phenomenon of grief seems to be the price of something that we would not live without, *viz.* love.

Apart from in existential writings (most significantly Kierkegaard's), it is difficult to find remnants of explicit articulations of the existential approach to suffering today. Those who (still) subscribe to this way of understanding and doing suffering are perhaps unlikely to articulate it explicitly, but it still exists rather more implicitly in certain parts of the world that have so far resisted the ever-growing therapy culture (Furedi, 2004). In my own country it is my impression that rural communities, in particular, still sometimes embody an ethos of stoicism and an acceptance of the hardships of life to a greater extent than people in urban areas. This, however, is difficult to assess, and one should beware of romanticizing these matters. On a more global scale, however, we have some evidence that the Western pathologization of people's reactions to traumatic events, such as the 2004 tsunami in Asia, sits uneasily with local social practices of coping with such disasters (Watters, 2010). There are still communities in which one turns to friends, neighbours and elders for help and advice on how to rebuild one's life, relationships, and house when facing existential turmoil, without a need for professional counsellors, therapists, or psychiatrists. We thus find across the world's cultures a variety of local practices and rituals for dealing with existential suffering, including emotional, social, and material support, but they typically and largely function in tacit and implicit ways.

The Moral Language

Notwithstanding the fact that the moral narrative is one of Shweder's "Big three", it might seem odd to include the moral language among the resources for making sense of suffering. In the West, we have become used to thinking of morality as a very narrow slice of human life that has to do only with evaluations of individual actions in light of moral values. However, in a broader sense, morality has to do with the "oughtness" of life as such: all the ways that normativity permeates our doings and sufferings (Brinkmann, 2011a). One obvious and important link between morality and suffering is represented by the moral emotions such as guilt and shame, both of which can be extremely painful. Through guilt, we experience having done something wrong, and through shame we feel the negative evaluation of the community of our selves (even if it is only imagined). Looked at through a diagnostic lens, however, such phenomena are quickly transformed into psychiatric conditions. If, for example, someone has acted immorally, say, has had an extra-marital affair, and subsequently suffers from a guilty conscience, ruminates and worries, develops negative automatic thoughts, and perhaps in consequence changes patterns of sleeping and eating, that person is very likely to score extremely high on most standard depression tests. However, at least from a common sense perspective, the person in question does not have a psychiatric problem, but rather a moral one. In order to be able to distinguish one from the other, it seems to be important to maintain a moral language of suffering, for merely counting symptoms will not do the trick.

More dramatic examples of clashes between moral and psychiatric languages can be found in jurisprudence, particularly when assessing whether someone is fit for the rule of law as in cases where the insanity defence is brought into play (Robinson, 1996). A famous recent case was the trial, in Norway, of Anders Behring Breivik, the far-right terrorist who killed 77 people in two attacks in 2011. The first psychiatric assessment concluded that he was a paranoid schizophrenic who suffered from psychotic delusions because of his belief that he was a knight of a Templar organization. A second assessment, however, declared that he was not psychotic, but suffered from anti-social and narcissistic personality disorders, which made him fit for legal punishment.[1]

If we move from examples to the principal discussion itself, we can say that there is a vital difference between the ways we can explain and understand human actions psychiatrically on the one hand, and morally on the other (see Brinkmann, 2013b). In the first case, we typically invoke a causal perspective, while the latter involves reference to reasons. If we ask: "Why did Jack and Jill go up the hill?", an explanation in terms of causes can state that they did so because their brains initiated a reaction in the locomotive system that made their legs move (a physiological explanation), because their genes wanted to replicate themselves in organisms known as offspring (a sociobiological explanation), or because they were forced to go up there by an inner demon (a psychiatric explanation that invokes a psychotic symptom, which was first judged to be the case in the Breivik trial). However different these are (and they need not rule one another out), they are all species of causal explanation that frame the situation as *behaviour* rather than *action*. The "behaviour", in this context, designates that something simply *happens* as a consequence of some mechanism (in the brain, genes, or body) that is either working well or in a pathological way, but without invoking meaning or normativity. However, we may also say that Jack and Jill went up the hill, because they wanted to smell the daisies. In this case, we understand the episode, not as a causal happening, but as human *action* that is based on a *reason* and an *intention* and expresses *meaning* (as Jack and Jill have heard that the hill is full of daisies and wish to experience the scent of these wonderful flowers). In this case, we conceive of Jack and Jill as agents that can act for a reason and to some extent articulate the reason that individuates their action (thereby *accounting* for their action). In addition, we may hold the actors responsible for what they have done; that is, praise or blame them (Robinson, 2002). It is difficult to imagine what human life would be like if we had no recourse to a language of reasons, and of praise and blame, also in relation to suffering and distress. It seems impossible to uphold an understanding of ourselves or others as agents without a normative language of reasons. According to MacIntyre, an understanding of what others are doing emerges only through ascribing reasons to them (MacIntyre, 1999). The moral language is thus important because it builds on a fundamental perspective

---

1 The details are well-described on Wikipedia: https://en.wikipedia.org/wiki/Anders_ Behring_Breivik.

on humans as *persons*, who are uniquely capable of giving and receiving reasons for action.

The discussion of reasons versus causes is enormous in philosophy, but I will here simply highlight three aspects that I find important in characterizing moral reason-giving: (1) that there is a primacy of reasons over causes in explanations of human action, (2) that reasons, unlike causes, are intransitive, and (3) that reasons are particularistic. As Hollis (1977) has argued regarding the first point, it seems to be the case that reasons are generally enough to explain actions. If a person does something and we are provided with a reason that satisfactorily explains the action, then the search for explanation normally stops. Only *irrational* actions call for causal explanations; that is, if we cannot find a *reason*-able explanation as to why someone did something. Furthermore, unlike causes, reasons are not transitive: if A is the cause of B, and B is the cause of C, then A is the cause of C. However, this does not go for reasons, for if A is the reason for my action B, then I am responsible for B, but I am not similarly responsible "for what others do autonomously because of what I set in motion" (p. 108). Responsibility and other moral concepts are not transitive in a simple way like causality. Finally, causes-explanations work by bringing particular observations under a general law, but reasons-explanations work differently, *viz.* by explaining "the particular by the particular" (p. 108). In general people do not act because their actions are instances of a general causal law. (For example, I do not love my wife because there is a general law specifying that humans of type x are attracted to humans of type y, but because she is lovable!) Even if there *is* a general law, this is not the *reason* why we act as we do.

If we relate these general considerations to the theme of pathologization, we can say that pathologizing some action often means suspending our common reason-giving practices and reinterpreting the action in light of a causal explanation. This can involve understanding the individual's behaviour as an instance of a general law ("this is what ADHD patients generally do"), or even invoking some causal mechanism in explaining a given occurrence ("it was the ADHD that caused him to..."), rather than invoking particularistic circumstances that render the action meaningful. This form of pathologizing can be, but need not be, driven by forces outside of the individual, but sometimes individuals are themselves active participants in processes of self-pathologization (such as in the process recently identified as ADHD-adoption, when undiagnosed individuals spread the word that they have ADHD; see Singh, 2011, and the following chapter).

Using Taylor's distinction introduced above, between explicit, symbolic and embodied aspects of understanding, in relation to *moral* suffering, we can conclude that explicitly, there are few social representations of this way of rendering suffering meaningful. The moral narrative lives, as Shweder's research has also shown, in many corners of the world, but most often in embodied and implicit social practices of giving reasons for the ways that people feel and act. Historically, however, the moral language has been much more influential on explicit levels, when people's sufferings and eccentricities were seen as moral defects, requiring moral therapy. But even today, I suspect that most of us intuitively feel that it is important to maintain a moral language that enables us, at least sometimes, to hold people responsible for their sufferings (in relation to acts that call for guilt or shame, for example). Where to draw the line between moral and causal understandings of misery will probably remain a crucial question in the years to come, not least because of the pressure that psychiatric diagnoses exert on national health systems, giving people access to benefits when a diagnosis reduces their personal responsibility (Williams, 2009).

The Political Language

Politics is a domain of our social life, where we struggle for and over rights, rules and goods. In a democracy, political processes are ideally organized so that all citizens are capable of being heard and can affect the decisions that are made. When citizens experience social injustice, for example, marginalization, disenfranchisement, discrimination or violations of rights, it is relevant to express one's disapproval in a political language. Traditionally, this language has been collective in the sense that political arguments are seen as legitimate to the extent that they refer to the rights and interests of the citizenry as a whole (or at least large groups such as workers, women etc.) rather than to specific individuals. It is not a legitimate political move – in a normative sense – to strive to change the law so that I benefit from it; one must argue that it is fair to change the law so that the conditions of my group are improved (for example, the rights of university professors).

In recent years, however, some analysts have argued that political language is gradually being transformed into a diagnostic language. Mary Boyle (2011) has argued that this is a process of "making the world go away", which converts "distress and problem behaviours to 'symptoms' and 'disorders'" (Boyle, 2011, p. 28). As a result, there is a grave risk of overlooking the fact that poverty, unemployment, marginalization, and so on, are very often the cause of (what is allegedly) "mental disorder" rather than consequences of it. Viewing people's lives through a diagnostic lens de-politicizes their problems and turns them into a matter of personal health and illness, to be treated pharmacologically or therapeutically (Smail, 2011). To give just one example, we might mention the "work stress epidemic", which has led to a wave of therapists, coaches and mindfulness instructors acting on employees and individuals, but with the risk of ignoring the roles of socio-material environments on people's lives (Wainwright & Calnan, 2002). Detrimental work conditions were once something to be dealt with politically and collectively – centred on the work of unions – but today are increasingly met with an individualizing and pathologizing response. Hermann and Kristensen pinpoint this development and argue that while workers used to engage in strike action collectively in order to protest against debilitating work conditions, people under individualized late-modern capitalism are left with the option of being sick with stress (Hermann & Kristensen, 2005). A political process has turned pathological and emotional, which might be a more general tendency in what Eva Illouz has termed an age of "emotional capitalism" (Illouz, 2007).

Politics, of course, is a huge and heterogeneous field with many explicit (for example, ideologies), symbolic (for example, ritualized meetings and demonstrations), and embodied (for example, feelings of injustice) levels of understanding. There is no danger that politics as such will disappear, but, if the analysis here has validity, there is a risk that those aspects of human suffering that were formerly articulated in a political language of rights and duties, social justice and injustice, will increasingly be addressed in individualized and diagnostic terms, thereby covering over the social backgrounds to human suffering.

Languages of Suffering and Possibilities for Action

After reviewing the languages of suffering that I have singled out as important, I will now address some of the possibilities for action that the different languages – and their associated social practices – enable for persons. But first it might be useful to remind ourselves of how varied the landscape of suffering and distress actually is.

In a discussion of mental disorder and its personal meanings, Bolton makes a distinction between three kinds of human distress, of which the kind that results from mental disorder is only one (Bolton, 2010). In addition to *pathological* distress, we have the kind of distress that is connected to normal *life transitions* (for example, in work, education, or family contexts), and distress connected to various forms of *social deprivation or exclusion*. From the analyses of the languages of suffering above, it is quite obvious that different languages are suitable for articulating different kinds of distress. A political language is most obviously connected to the third category mentioned by Bolton – intent, as it is, on thematizing processes of power and social (un)justice – whereas a moral language is often relevant in relation to life transitions (a divorce, for example, may be the result of one party's deceitful behaviour), which can also be said of the existential language (relevant, for example, in relation to experiences of loss). Like the diagnostic language, the religious language can be a colonizing language that seeks to dominate the understanding of suffering, which happens when all the problems that befall humans (from physical illness to poverty) are interpreted as the reactions of an almighty deity to the sinful actions of human beings. On a less "imperialist" reading, however, the religious language can be said, like the existential and moral languages, to concern itself with making suffering meaningful by placing it within a cosmic framework, or what Taylor has called an *ontic logos* (Taylor, 1989).

One way to take the analysis of the present chapter is to engage in further cultural critique of the imperialist tendencies of the current diagnostic language, which is something that is addressed throughout this book. Quite another way concerns the normative question of when to use a given language. How do we in fact know when to use a given language in relation to a specific instance of human distress? How do we know when, say, my diffuse sense of sadness and emptiness is clinical depression (diagnostic language), and when it is my human response to mortality and sin (religious language), an expression of existential despair (existential language), a manifestation of guilty conscience (moral language), or a sign of stress felt when working in a socially accelerating late modern world (political language)? These are different hermeneutic readings of the same "symptoms" (psychological and physical) that enable different aspects of one's situation to appear as salient. Different opportunities for action will also appear in the process of interpretation, and pragmatists will insist that the question is not simply that of deciding which of the languages is the *correct* one (according to a correspondence theory of truth), but concerns which one of the languages leads to *fruitful* consequences in terms of actions and experiences.

Continuing on the pragmatist note, we can say that the different languages offer the suffering person different subject positions; that is, involve different forms of positioning. (See Harré, Moghaddam, Cairnie, Rothbart & Sabat, 2009, for a recent exposition of positioning theory.) To simplify, we can say that the diagnostic language in some cases will position the person as a patient, literally as a passive site of psychiatric dysfunctions (possibly rooted in the brain) that happen to affect the person in detrimental ways. Given this perspective, one is not as such an agent, but a location in a chain of causal processes. However, in other cases, the diagnostic language may also lead to externalizations of the person's problems in a way that actually does position the person as agent; that is, as active in relation to "coping" with his or her problems through the diagnostic framing and all that follows from a diagnosis (for example, access to patient organizations, psychoeducation, and problem-solving exercises in everyday life). The point is, however, that the resources for this kind of active positioning through the diagnostic language must come from outside the diagnostic language itself. In itself, the diagnostic language is one of causes and effects rather than one of persons and actions. So, in order to enable an active positioning, the diagnostic language must look in particular to existential and moral resources, which "specialize" in agential language. The argument here is analogous to Harré's argument that understanding others through the Person-grammar, thus positioning them as persons that perform meaningful acts and can articulate reasons for action, is and ought to be primary over grammars (languages or vocabularies) that approach others as organisms (O-grammar) or clusters of molecules (M-grammar) (Harré, 2002). This is foundational for the person centred cultural psychological perspective of this book. The reductive languages are not useless or redundant just because they are reductive, for they are important conceptual resources that enable us to address vital features of human beings – but, and this is an important but, they are necessarily parasitic on a more fundamental understanding of others as *persons*. (Harré develops this into the so-called Taxonomic Priority Principle, which states that we can only approach something as an organismic or molecular aspect of a psychological process – such as depression – once it has been identified as a process experienced or enacted by persons.) Likewise, the diagnostic language is parasitic on those languages that position others as acting persons and articulate suffering as something that can, at least in principle, be a meaningful response to the world's events. It seems to be that only when no reasons are within discursive reach should we turn to causal explanations. Sadly, however, the ways that the diagnostic language is used is one that often conceals this very fact, thereby giving us something like the two-dimensional view of life described by Healy at the beginning of this chapter.

There is thus a risk of blocking the necessary understanding of persons having agency, if the diagnostic language becomes hegemonic in relation to human suffering. However, there is also the adverse risk of positioning the person as an agent in relation to matters that are completely outside that person's control. This has been discussed but little in the literature that is critical of diagnostic psychiatry, but it can in fact be detrimental to human well-being if one is addressed as an agent in relation to "non-agential" issues, which is to say, matters beyond one's control. Thus, there might be a limit to pragmatism in a sense: the strength of pragmatism lies in its idea that the language we use, and the kinds of positioning involved, can lead to human growth and development toward greater autonomy and enhanced agency. But not *any* kind of positioning is realistic, and an overly "optimistic" form of agential positioning may even lead to new problems for the persons involved, as they risk blaming themselves for their inadequacies (following the logic that "If I am a free agent with the capacity of choosing, and yet I am still suffering, then I must be the one to blame", which may lead to worsened suffering and so on in a vicious cycle of blaming the victim). That is why, to put it somewhat schematically, we must supplement the pragmatic interest in action possibilities (afforded by different languages inherent in social practices) with a hermeneutic interest in interpreting the person and her suffering in her life situation as it presents itself in its "facticity" (to borrow a term from Heidegger). In relation to this, we should also bear in mind that the question of languages, and which one to use, is rarely a matter of "either-or". In practice, different languages often work simultaneously in people's self-understandings, and most people are not only capable of tolerating this, but also benefit from it. A person diagnosed with ADHD may thus invoke one language in conversations with a psychiatrist, and other languages when meeting employers, friends and family, for example. A certain kind of linguistic flexibility is often at play, and the languages of suffering, including the diagnostic one, do not determine people's self-understandings mechanically.

At least one hugely important conclusion for mental health professionals follows from this: there seems to be no way of outsourcing judgments about when to use which language in relation to a given suffering person. No algorithm or manual seems capable of doing the trick, for these (for example, the diagnostic tests) presuppose that the judgment concerning which language to use has already been made. Simply diagnosing various forms of human suffering through tests and symptom checklists thus misses the process of understanding and analyzing the situated, contextual particulars that are often crucial. What is worse, it may lead to the blocking of otherwise fertile developmental pathways for persons if they come to appropriate a misleading language when articulating their problems, for example, one that positions them as passive patients of symptoms rather than acting persons.

Conclusions

So far, I have in this book introduced diagnostic cultures and articulated a cultural psychological framework that is relevant when studying processes in this cultural situation. We have seen how psychiatric diagnoses can be approached as epistemic objects, and I have discussed their problematic status as natural kinds. In this chapter, I have looked directly at the diagnostic language of suffering that is prevalent today and drawn a number of contrasts to other significant languages of suffering. In the next chapter, I shall give an account of how diagnoses function as semiotic mediators in the lives of those who are diagnosed.

Chapter 4
Psychiatric Diagnoses as Semiotic Mediators

As we saw at the beginning of this book, historically, as well as in contemporary social science, psychiatry has been heavily criticized. Thomas Szasz (1961) famously argued that the very concept of 'mental illness' is a myth and should be discarded; Erving Goffman and others following in his footsteps tried to demonstrate empirically that psychiatric practices were inhumane and stigmatizing (Goffman, 1961); and more recent critics have argued that current conceptions of mental illness/disorder are overinclusive and pathologizing (Wakefield, 2010), and that the medical industry makes people's lives worse because of the debilitating long-term side-effects of drug treatments (Healy, 2012; Whitaker, 2010). Although these critical analyses are all worth discussing, and all have something to contribute in the current age that is seemingly dominated by various psychiatric epidemics (ranging from stress, depression and anxiety to ADHD and personality disorders) and a general "medicalization of society" (Conrad, 2007), they do not capture the significant experience of being diagnosed, or the various roles that psychiatric diagnoses play in the lives of the diagnosed today. In the words of Comstock, who has recently been charting the genealogy of the ADHD subject:

> the conventional critical perspectives fail to account for how it is possible that so many would accept being controlled or 'drugged' within broad trends of 'over-diagnosis' except by simplifying (or denying) the role of the individual in subjectification through the worn out critical concepts 'ideology' and 'social control'. (Comstock, 2011, p. 49)

What was analyzed by the anti-psychiatric movement from the 1960s onwards as oppressive ideology and social control (working through stigmatizing unwanted behaviours as mental illness), appears in the 21st century as something that is often actively sought by people, who may be looking for conceptual resources with which to explain their problems and render their suffering meaningful. How, then, do people use a psychiatric diagnosis in relation to their own lives and experienced problems? And how can a diagnosis function as a resource for self-understanding? These questions are addressed in the present chapter.

The chapter delves into the diagnostic cultures of adults diagnosed with ADHD (particularly as the diagnostic culture emerges in a support group) to study how this diagnosis comes to function as a filter through which people interpret their problems, or as a resource that is used both unreflectively and reflectively to mediate people's actions and emotions. (Gillespie & Zittoun, 2010, introduce a helpful distinction between mediation and reflective use of tools and signs, but, in this chapter, I refer to both processes as mediation.) The psychiatric language has been democratized in the sense that it has entered everyday conversations about people's problems. We know *that* diagnoses (here the ADHD diagnosis) are increasingly used as semiotic mediators, but too often researchers draw simplistic conclusions about this. Sometimes, they claim that the use of the diagnostic language as a resource is itself therapeutic (Wykes & Callard, 2010, p. 301), possibly because of its potential to "externalize" people's problems), and sometimes it is claimed that diagnoses cultivate passivity and vulnerability (Furedi, 2004), or are downright iatrogenic, a view represented for example by Jutel (2011), who argues that the expansion of diagnostic categories "is not without risk and can have severe iatrogenic results" (p. 10) when people begin to interpret their problems as psychiatric afflictions, leading perhaps to unnecessary pharmaceutical remedies.

In this chapter, I aim to add nuances to, and qualify the discussion of, the effects of psychiatric diagnoses on individuals, by focusing on three specific functions that psychiatric diagnoses can have as semiotic mediators in people's lives in today's diagnostic cultures. First, diagnoses can be used in an *explanatory* way, which I argue is extremely widespread, although strictly speaking the explanatory function is circular. Second, diagnoses can be used in *self-affirming* ways; that is to say, as a filter that transforms numerous life phenomena into symptoms that come to affirm the diagnosis. And third, diagnoses can be used in disclaiming ways as constituting *exemption from responsibility*, whether this is warranted or not. I make no claims about the frequency of these uses of diagnoses, for I am only interested in charting and describing them analytically. My impression, however, is that all of them are very widespread in discursive practices involving the ADHD category and likely also with respect to other diagnoses.

My analysis is based on empirical materials collected as part of ongoing fieldwork in a support group for adults diagnosed with ADHD in Denmark. The group meets every month for about three hours, and I have followed the group for a couple of years now. In addition to participating in the group, I also conduct individual in-depth interviews with a smaller number of key informants, and I am furthermore engaged in analyses of the discourses and wider social representations of ADHD that circulate in both national and international media. By drawing upon these different sources of materials, the goal is to approach the ADHD diagnosis from many perspectives at the same time, to get a broad sense of the individual and cultural impact of this diagnosis. This chapter, however, develops its categories solely based on the fieldwork, since I am interested in how the participants here use ADHD as a semiotic mediator.

The ADHD Diagnosis

ADHD has become a well-known and much discussed diagnosis, and I have already referred to it a number of times in this book, but what is it? Quite a lot of research has been conducted with children diagnosed with ADHD, but so far much less concerning adults, which has led some to claim that the literature on this kind of ADHD diagnosis is almost non-existent (Comstock, 2011, p. 65). Today, most researchers acknowledge that ADHD persists into adulthood in about 60 per cent of the children diagnosed, thus affecting approximately four per cent of adults worldwide, according to authoritative estimates (Adler & Shaw, 2011). With broad screening criteria, one recognized study found a prevalence as high as 16.4 per cent in US adults (Faraone & Biederman, 2005). From the mainstream medical perspective, the core symptoms of ADHD are inattention, hyperactivity, and impulsivity, with the former being the most significant symptom for most adults who are diagnosed. ADHD is conventionally seen as a neurobiological disorder that is commonly treated with drugs (although no consensus has been reached regarding the precise nature of the neurological problem involved), and with a significant genetic component. The standard medical history of the diagnosis claims that ADHD has been with us for a long time, albeit under different conceptual guises, and many textbooks begin their accounts with the German physician Heinrich Hoffman, who described "Fidgety Philip" in 1844, and the English pediatrician George Still, who published his observations of hyperactive children in *The Lancet* in 1902, although on closer scrutiny it becomes unclear whether these early researchers actually described what we think of as ADHD today (Smith, 2012, p. 26). Hyperactivity has been referred to with many different terms in the course of history, culminating with the ADHD diagnosis finally being established as late as 1987 in DSM-III-R.

Many other approaches besides the medical one have been taken towards ADHD, such as sociological ones arguing that diagnosing ADHD is a species of medicalization and social control (Conrad, 2006), and also historical ones that point to features of American society as providing a niche for the diagnostic birth and expansion of ADHD (Smith, 2012). Borrowing from Hacking's (2006) terminology, we can say that some scholars are *sceptics* and argue that it (*in casu* ADHD, but similar discussions exist for other psychiatric diagnoses) has never existed and that the diagnosis has always been specious (this being the critical position in the literature); others are *enthusiasts* and argue that it has always existed, even before the diagnostic category emerged (this is probably the majority view, represented by most medical approaches to ADHD).

Although my ambition in this chapter is not to discuss the ontology of the ADHD phenomenon, I should probably say that I find both of these approaches to be simplifying and caught in an unhelpful dilemma. Following Hacking, I believe that the most fruitful approach is one that analyzes ADHD as a real phenomenon, although bearing in mind that its reality depends on certain sociocultural niches and practices. Another way to put it has been articulated by Mol, who argues that diseases (she studied atherosclerosis, but her approach seems even more to the point in relation to psychiatric entities) are not so much "constructed" as they are *done, performed*, or *enacted* in and through cultural practices (Mol, 2002). Like Mol, the kind of cultural psychology articulated in this book favours a "praxiographic appreciation of reality" (p. 53), according to which social and psychological phenomena are not only *had* and *experienced*, but also *done* by skilled human actors, mediated by a host of material and symbolic devices (Brinkmann, 2011b; see also Chapter 7). Emphasizing enactment and doing, Mol asks: "Who does the doing?" and the answer is *not* isolated individuals, for "Events are made to happen by several people and lots of things. Words participate, too. Paperwork. Rooms, buildings. The insurance system. An endless list of heterogeneous elements" (Mol, 2002, pp. 25–26). I do not have space to unfold a full cultural-praxiographic analysis of ADHD in this chapter, but will limit myself to throwing light on how the diagnostic category itself is actively used by some of the adults diagnosed (keeping in mind that what they do with this category is closely interwoven with many other cultural practices and preconditions).

Using a Diagnosis as Semiotic Mediator

As I will discuss in this text, people – including patients diagnosed – use psychiatric diagnoses as semiotic mediators for different purposes and with different results. That diagnoses travel widely, including outside the systems they were created for, is a pervasive cultural phenomenon. According to Pickersgill, the DSM today functions as a "connective tissue" on a large cultural scale for many different groups with a stake in psychiatry (Pickersgill, 2012, p. 331). In that sense, the psychiatric diagnoses have become very significant boundary objects in the contemporary West; that is, objects of knowledge which "inhabit several communities of practice and satisfy the informational requirements of each of them" (Bowker & Star, 2000, p. 16).

What ADHD is, for example, is on the one hand a "something" that is sufficiently stable across communities of practice, as defined in the diagnostic manuals, but on the other is polyvalent in its meanings for children, parents, teachers, doctors, researchers, the medical industry, the public, and so on. The diagnoses are categories that connect these very different sets of actors and their communities of practice, and focus actors' attention on certain properties highlighted as problematic, although this does not necessarily happen in harmonious or homogenous ways (Brinkmann, 2014a). With this broader cultural network of actors and practices organized through diagnostic categories in mind, I now move on to the local understandings manifested by members of the ADHD support group.

During the first meeting I attended in the ADHD support group, I was given a very clear indication of the dominant discourse of ADHD in this community. The meetings always begin with a round of presentations. Each participant (there are normally 10–15 people at a meeting with a mix of newcomers and regulars) introduces him or herself, and is supposed to inform the others about something positive that has happened since the previous meeting. Quite often, however, the presentations move from positive stories into accounts of negative and problematic experiences, especially in relation to encounters with "the system", which comprises general practitioners, psychiatrists, and representatives of the welfare state (counsellors and social workers). The other participants provide emotional support and encouragement, and also often give practical advice concerning how to navigate personal, legal, or medical issues.

I was given my first impression of the dominant discourse when Thomas (all names and identifying details are changed) presented himself and began by saying: "I've had ADHD for four years". Immediately, other participants in the group interrupted and corrected him. One of them, Joanna, said: "No, Thomas, your ADHD was *discovered* four years ago. You have always had ADHD, right?" Thomas nodded and laughed, and it became evident that this group considers ADHD a congenital disorder. The group is organized by the Danish ADHD association (www.adhd.dk), which is sponsored by various pharmaceutical companies such as Eli Lilly. This association parallels the US patient organization CHADD (www.chadd.org), and works with an understanding of ADHD as a neurobiological disorder with a significant genetic component that should be treated with drugs. The group conversations are moderated by a person, who does not have the diagnosis, but is engaged in voluntary work in the association (his son is diagnosed with ADHD, he told me, which motivates him to help others). The moderator visibly relates to the ADHD association through various forms of merchandise, for instance, a bag with an ADHD logo.

Regardless of the truth value of the biomedical understanding of ADHD, it has a number of effects on how the diagnosis is used to mediate the self-understanding of those diagnosed, which has also been found by other researchers (Halleröd, Anckarsäter, Råstam & Scherman, 2015). This is probably less pervasive in children than in adults, who have often actively sought a diagnosis by contacting their doctor or psychiatrist (after their children have received the diagnosis, for example). A typical story is that the adults have felt different from others for a long time, but without being able to explain why. This takes us to the first kind of semiotic mediation that the ADHD diagnosis is involved in, which I here call explanatory mediation.

Explanatory Mediation

The ADHD diagnosis is used in an explanatory way by almost all participants in the group at some point. They typically invoke ADHD as an explanation when they summarize their life stories (when they introduce themselves to newcomers in the group, for example). Mike's account is typical: he lives alone with his dog (and the dog figures in many of his stories and is clearly very important to him, not least because of its capacity to calm him down when he becomes aggressive), and he otherwise experiences numerous problems with social relationships. He explains that his problem is that he "snaps" easily and can become quite violent, especially towards representatives of the welfare system, but, as he says, "When I received the diagnosis, I finally got an explanation why I snap". ADHD as a diagnosis mediates Mike's understanding of his own problematic behaviours, and is used as an explanation.

Another story is Marie's. She has experienced numerous problems in her life, which culminated when she became a mother: "For several years, I just played computer games. I was addicted, and I couldn't get up and get my daughter to school." She referred to the diagnostic process as a "revelation" that changed her life: "There is my life before the diagnosis and after the diagnosis. I still hit the ground once in a while, but today I know *why!*" Again, the diagnosis is used to explain her problematic patterns of behaviour. This is so widespread that it initially escaped my attention, but when I discovered it, I observed it again and again. It also figures in some of the official ADHD documents and plans in Denmark, for example, in the ADHD strategy formulated by the municipality of Aarhus (the second largest city in Denmark). This text repeats several times that the ADHD diagnosis "provides the individual with an explanation of the troubles he or she encounters" (Aarhus Kommune, 2013, p. 4; my translation). Other researchers have also noticed how receiving an ADHD diagnosis gives relief through providing an explanation. In an interview study with 8 adults diagnosed, Young and colleagues report: "Immediately after their diagnosis, participants described an initial sense of relief and elation that their lifelong quest for an explanation had finally come to an end" (Young, Bramham, Gray, & Rose, 2008, p. 496). However, the authors add that this relief is typically short-lived and is followed by new feelings of confusion, something which is also articulated by several of my informants.

As Wilkinson has argued, people engage in struggles to bestow meaning upon suffering not just as an intellectual endeavour, but as part of psychic healing (Wilkinson, 2005, p. 18). It is bad enough to suffer, but if one's suffering appears as lacking in meaning, it is even worse, so humans look for explanations that change the meaningless into something meaningful, and the whole diagnostic system has today become significant in this regard as an explanatory "language of suffering" (Brinkmann, 2014a). The problem with this, however, is that it is circular. In the case of ADHD, the diagnosis cannot be formulated on the basis of biomarkers (for example, blood samples or brain scans), but only by counting and evaluating symptoms, as they appear on various symptom checklists, for instance. The circularity emerges when the diagnosis is formulated with reference to problematic behaviours, and the same behaviours are explained with reference to the diagnosis. First, the person is identified (either by himself or herself or others) as problematic, perhaps because of impulsivity or inattention, and seeks help or gathers information from various sources (notably the internet). Second, if the problems are severe enough to count as symptoms of ADHD, this diagnosis is formulated to account for the problematic behaviours. Finally, if one asks how we know that ADHD is in fact the problem, the answer is that this is evident from the symptoms (Timimi, 2009). The symptoms thus warrant the diagnostic category, which is in turn invoked to explain the symptoms in a circular, and ultimately empty, process. This circular process goes on both intramentally, so to speak, in the diagnosed person's own understanding of her predicament, and intermentally in the person's relationship with medical and social authorities, which often also use the diagnosis explanatorily.

Although the participants in the support group use the ADHD category as a way of explaining their problems, they are not directly aware of the inbuilt circularity, but it might nonetheless affect them indirectly, for example, when people around them fail to understand their problems. The societal discussion about ADHD (both in Denmark, but also in many other countries) often concerns the lack of "objective" ways of formulating the diagnosis. Almost all participants say that they enjoy being in the group, because no one questions their diagnosis so they do not have to be defensive. They meet suspicion in many other corners of their life, when they have to shield themselves against charges that their problems are no bigger than anyone else's. Mark says that the worst thing about telling others of his ADHD and problems with impulsivity and inattention is when people respond: "Well, I know that from myself", tacitly implying that he is no worse off than other people without the diagnosis (and many other group participants express a similar attitude).

Using ADHD in a process of explanatory mediation often involves a kind of "entification" of the problematic behaviours (Valsiner, 2007). Entification involves transforming a trait, temperament, emotion or some other psychological phenomenon into a "thing", typically with alleged causal powers to affect action, and it is this process that makes explanatory mediation work as a process, for often there has to be some "harmful agent" inside the diagnosed that can be categorized, if the diagnosis is to count as an explanation – however circular it may be. The discourse in the group is full of entification in the sense that members continuously talk about "my ADHD" and "what my ADHD does". For example, as Marie explains: "My ADHD makes me forget my appointments, so I have to tell my friends to call me just before I am going to meet them". ADHD becomes a "something" within the person that acts on the person, often in detrimental ways. Without wanting to compare ADHD to demonic possession in other ways, the parallel regarding entification is nonetheless interesting. As Littlewood has pointed out in a comparison of "Western" conceptions of psychiatric disease entities with "indigenous" ideas of spirit possession:

> Professional intervention in a sickness involves incorporating the patient into an overarching system of explanation, a common structural pattern which manifests itself in the bodily economy of every human being. Accountability is transferred onto an agency beyond the patient's control: diseases now rather than the spirits. (Littlewood, 2002, p. 48)

Entification involves the discursive creation of some agent within the person that causes the problem, and this goes on in a dynamic process between individuals, who are invited into this process by the prevalent public discourses about ADHD. Schmitz and colleagues studied the social representations of ADHD in the media and found that there is a process of "anchoring" and "objectification" so that "uncertainty about the causal aspects of ADHD became anchored in a physical illness depiction through the scientific findings using brain-imaging technology", and this was objectified through the media's use of terms such as "'broken brain', 'brakes off brains' and 'derailed concentration'" (Schmitz, Filippone, & Edelman, 2003, p. 400). The scientific brain discourse ("brainism") is here translated into the vernacular and is used by people as an explanation through entification (the "broken brain" and similar expressions serving as relevant causal entities, although none of the group members' brains have been examined).

Self-affirming Mediation

What I have called explanatory mediation is a key function of the ADHD diagnosis for the members of the group, and can be considered the fundamental one, but two other and probably subordinate ways that the diagnosis mediates the members' understanding of their affliction should be noted here. First, we have self-affirming mediation. With this term, I refer to the tendency of the diagnosis to affirm itself, not only because numerous phenomena become "symptoms" when seen through the diagnostic lens (which has often been noted by critical social scientists who emphasize the danger of everyday problems being pathologized through diagnoses), but also because even phenomena in a person's life that could be expected to *count against* the ADHD diagnosis are affirmed as the very expression of it.

Various examples from the fieldwork could be used as illustrations here, but I shall mention just a few. William talks about his life and his problems and says that he "likes very much to keep everything in order to avoid the chaos". Like others in the group, he is extremely structured with checklists and engages in tidying up. What is interesting is that he mentions this as an example of how his ADHD manifests itself, although the diagnostic category is often associated with forgetfulness and a disordered life (a key diagnostic criterion is that people have difficulties organizing tasks and activities). Mark's story is similar. Mark very much identifies with the ADHD diagnosis. He is a resourceful person that helps others in the group (with medication and contact with "the system", for example), and he has the letters A D H D tattooed on his chest. Like William, Mark is extremely organized, and he has worked in various store houses, which suited him perfectly because he could work professionally to keep order. He has what he calls "benign OCD" in addition to his ADHD, and "the two keep each other in check", as he says, again invoking a form of entification with two forces struggling within him. However, it is interesting that a trait of orderliness that many would see as praiseworthy is mentioned as a symptom of the disorder. This is what I call self-affirmation. Once the diagnosis has been made, both phenomena that could previously have counted for as well as against the diagnosis are used by the diagnosed to affirm the diagnosis. Had William and Mark *not* lived an orderly life (as is the case with others in the group, who invoke this problem as a symptom of ADHD), this could also have been used to affirm the diagnosis. One is reminded of the classic critique of psychoanalysis that it is non-falsifiable, because whatever interpretation the analyst makes of the patient can be construed as valid – for if the patient agrees, the interpretation is confirmed, and if she disagrees, it is likewise confirmed, because it is a sure sign that she is in denial! The ADHD entity construed within (and by) the person clearly works in different, and sometimes contradictory, ways.

Disclaiming Mediation

Finally, I shall address the way that the ADHD diagnosis is used to mediate a self-understanding that disclaims responsibility. Again, this can be seen as a subcategory of the explanatory function, since responsibility is often transferred from the person as a volitional subject and onto the "ADHD entity", as I discussed above with reference to entification. A typical example of how the diagnosis is used to disclaim responsibility is found in Marie's statements (referring to what happened when she was diagnosed) that, "the worst thing my psychiatrist could say was that there was nothing wrong with me. In that case, I was simply lazy, you know!" A similar concern was expressed by Michelle, a young woman who lives with her boyfriend on whom she depends a lot, since she does not like to be in her house by herself – something she sees as related to her diagnosed ADHD. In her job, she has informed her manager of her diagnosis in order to explain why she is sometimes unable to get things done. Finally, Mark mentioned how he often reacts without thinking, for example, when an elderly woman took hold of his son's arm in a zoo, scolding him (because the boy threw small stones), and Mark reacted by grabbing her arm violently and verbally abusing her. He explained that this was not him reacting, but the ADHD within him, and that he is now trying to learn to control his aggressive behaviour by noticing how his frustration builds up from a warm sensation in the back of his neck, leading him to say to himself, "Now, my ADHD is taking over", and he tries to remove himself from the problematic situation.

That the ADHD diagnosis can be used disclaimingly in relation to responsibility and common moral demands has been noted in the literature, and, in her study of ADHD children, Singh reports that almost all the children diagnosed with ADHD (in a UK sample) said they had used ADHD as an excuse (Singh, 2011, p. 894). Perhaps it is this feature of the diagnosis that leads to a new phenomenon observed by Singh, *viz.* what she calls "ADHD-adoption", which is when undiagnosed people "spread the word that they have ADHD in order to build up their personal armament against harassment, thereby further instantiating the stereotype" (p. 894). If "is it not me" who is acting in non-desirable ways, but this something in me – ADHD – then I am not to blame, for the disorder is the true agent. It is understandable that this can be an attractive self-understanding, even for people who are not diagnosed, because it removes (or at least lessens) the burden of moral fault. If responsibility is central to human concerns, however, then there are problems with this medicalization of morality, but a more positive aspect should also be noted, as we saw in Mark's story before: the diagnosis can be invoked as a semiotic mediator that enables the person to distance himself from his own aggression and frustration, leading to a conflict becoming downplayed, because the blame is conferred neither upon the ego, the person himself, nor upon the alter, the other person in a conflict (which was the elderly lady in the story told by Mark), but to the ADHD entity within, leading to increased personal control in this case.

ADHD Identity

What kind of person does one become when the ADHD diagnosis is used as a semiotic mediator of one's self-understanding? How can one have, be and do ADHD? No simple answer emerges from the analyses above, but it does seem that the diagnosis affords a self-understanding of oneself as "possessed" by some entity with powers to create problems in one's life. Referring to this entity in reflections and conversations with others can be used to *explain* the problems (explanatory mediation), while employing the diagnosis as a mediator has a tendency to *affirm* one's problems as stemming from ADHD, even in cases where the person copes or compensates quite well (self-affirming mediation). Finally, ADHD as a semiotic mediator can also be used as an *excuse* for oneself and others, thereby disclaiming responsibility (disclaiming mediation).

It should be noted that none of the group participants included in my study mediate their self-understanding exclusively through the ADHD diagnosis. Like all of us, they draw on numerous sources, languages and categories, but this chapter has singled out some of the significant ways that the diagnosis is used – and, needless to say, since the participants come together in the group precisely in order to help each other because of their ADHD, they are probably likely to invoke the diagnostic category much more in this setting than they otherwise would. I would also like to stress that there is no determinism involved, such that being diagnosed automatically leads to some kind of "ADHD identity"; rather, the diagnosis is used flexibly and creatively by skilled human actors for different purposes, which is why I here approach the diagnosis as an interpretative resource, a semiotic mediator (rather than a "causal variable") that affords (rather than determines) certain uses.

As I touched upon, there are significant theoretical problems in constructing an entity out of the ADHD diagnosis (entification), but these theoretical problems do not seem to bother the participants much in practice, for entification is an omnipresent feature of how the diagnosis is invoked when they talk about their lives and problems. However, I would like to propose the interpretation that indirectly, entification creates problems for the simple reason that no objective entity has been observed to which the diagnostic category refers. ADHD is a set of symptoms, and I discussed the circularity involved in the process whereby the symptoms are used to formulate the diagnosis that is in turn invoked to explain the symptoms. It is precisely the lack of "objective" criteria for the ADHD diagnosis that is perhaps the most important feature of the public criticism that the diagnosis meets. The lack of biomarkers has lead Joseph (among other critics) to conclude that "ADHD is simply a grouping of socially disapproved behaviours falsely passed off as a disease" (Joseph, 2009, p. 75). As I made clear earlier in the chapter, my goal in this context is not to establish whether ADHD is a "real disease" or not, or whether the diagnosis is valid or not, but rather to investigate how people use the diagnosis as a semiotic mediator in a diagnostic culture. However, the point here is that these issues cannot be completely separated, since the participants partly use the category as a resource in ways that sometimes reflect, and sometimes go against, the public discussions of ADHD.

Semiotic Mediation of Other Psychiatric Categories

Although the focus of the present chapter is ADHD, it can be noted that other researchers are now studying how other psychiatric or quasi-psychiatric categories semiotically mediate people's relationships to themselves and their suffering. One example is found in the work of Ester Holte Kofod, who investigates current conceptualizations and experiences of grief, particularly as this phenomenon (like many others) is undergoing medicalization and possibly pathologization with the introduction of diagnostic labels for pathological grief such as persistent complex bereavement disorder, which was introduced into DSM-5's section III as a condition for further studies (Kofod, 2015). Many had expected (and critics had feared) that a proper official grief diagnosis would be ready for DSM-5, but this did not happen, and instead the bereavement exclusion for major depressive disorders was removed so that it is now possible to be diagnosed with depression two weeks after a loss. In light of these developments, Kofod studies how bereaved parents experience and practise their grief after infant loss. The study is a qualitative interview study, and Kofod has identified four main ways in which the parents relate to the possibility of having their grief diagnosed:

(1) Diagnosis as a legitimating practice – There is tendency among the bereaved parents to see a diagnosis as a possible legitimatization of their suffering. If they could obtain a grief diagnosis (which is currently not possible in Denmark) they can obtain emotional "advantages" ("to have the right to grieve"), material ones (such as access to sick leave, economic and therapeutic support) and also relational ones (since a diagnostic category might give them a legitimate way of communicating the suffering to others). Both in relation to family and workplace, the participants in the interview study report that a diagnosis would make it easier to communicate about their suffering and inability to perform their normal routines.

(2) Diagnosis as a demarcation practice – Among the majority of the participants there is the idea that a grief diagnosis could be used to differentiate between normal or natural reactions on the one hand and pathological or dysfunctional grief reactions on the other. Demarcations between normal and pathological grief

are made with reference to normative standards regarding the intensity, duration and content of emotional expressions: normal grieving allows for a certain degree and duration of emotional pain, while pathological grief is associated with prolonged, overly intense and negative emotional expressions like bitterness and anger (Kofod, 2015).

(3) Diagnosis as (illegitimate) pathologization – This third account counters all pathologization of grief and maintains that even intense and long-lasting grief ought to be considered as a normal reaction to a profound loss. This position is found among some of the participants, while the final one is represented by just one voice.

(4) Diagnosis as a normative ideal – This final account represents an intriguing challenge to the widely held notion of psychiatric diagnoses as stigmatizing, according to Kofod: one participant states that given the existence of a grief diagnosis, she would feel an urge to "live up to" the criteria in order to prove to herself (and others) that she loved her dead child. She says that if she did not get the diagnosis, she would ask: "Do I not grieve enough for my child?" Interestingly – and in some ways paradoxically – the formulation of diagnoses can articulate scripts for how to think, feel and act in various difficult life situations.

Grief is not (yet) an official psychiatric diagnosis, just as ADHD was not one until quite recently, but I have included a treatment of Kofod's work here because it demonstrates how people can also employ a quasi-diagnosis or border diagnosis to semiotically mediate a relationship to their suffering. As was the case with the ADHD diagnosis, a significant finding is that this does not happen in deterministic or universal ways, but is something flexible that people negotiate depending on many different factors and contextual features.

Conclusions

Having reviewed various ways that psychiatric diagnoses – in this case ADHD (with a brief reference to the border diagnosis of grief) – can be used by those diagnosed in order for them to understand their lives and regulate their actions, I shall in the next chapter move on to analyze more generally how psychiatric identity or subjectivity is constituted in our diagnostic cultures, not least through the use of quantitative measures. This also provides for a more macro sociological account of the current significance of psychiatric diagnoses.

Chapter 5
"Do More, Feel Better, Live Longer": Being a Psychiatric Subject

"Do more, feel better, live longer" is the slogan of GlaxoSmithKline, considered the second largest pharmaceutical company in the world. There is much to say about this company in relation to our diagnostic cultures. Among other things, it is infamous for recently paying a 3 billion dollar fine, mainly because of its illicit promotion of the antidepressants Wellbutrin and Paxil for unapproved uses. I shall not here pursue the negative stories about GlaxoSmithKline, nor shall I discuss the iatrogenic effects of long-term use of antidepressants. Much is being written at present about how the drugs can actually make people ill (and I return to this theme in the next chapter). Instead, I shall concern myself with the ideology, the culturally sanctioned life philosophy one could say, that the slogan of GlaxoSmithKline embodies and discuss how it relates to diagnostic cultures, and I shall argue that although this and other pharmaceutical companies have the explicit goal of fighting various psychopathologies, the approach to life inherent in the "do more, feel better, live longer" mentality actually amounts to something like a social pathology in itself, which is one engine in the promotion of the diagnostic language of suffering.

I follow Paterson in viewing advertising as "the poetry of capitalism" (Paterson, 2006), so, although a slogan such as this one might seem completely innocent, it actually brings forth a certain aesthetics and underlying logic concerning how one should live and think about life as a person in the 21st century. This is related, I shall argue, to the dominant views of psychiatric subjectivity today, found also in the logic of current diagnostics, which are by and large quantitative, but which thereby fail to understand the qualitative aspects of human self-identity, as articulated, for example, by Charles Taylor in the last couple of decades. I shall argue that the rush toward a quantified subjectivity – with psychiatric diagnoses playing a key role in the process – can be seen as an attempt to create a kind of solidity in an era that Zygmunt Bauman has otherwise addressed as liquid modernity.

The Quantified Self

Alongside the development of diagnostic cultures as addressed in this book, we have witnessed an increased quantification of the self or subject in psychiatric practices.[1]

---

1 I use the concepts "self" and "subject" ("selfhood" and "subjectivity") interchangeably in this context.

What is meant by a "quantitative" view of subjectivity? It is in fact quite easy to see in the psychopharmaceutical slogan "Do *more*, feel *better*, live *longer*", since these are all imperatives that lend themselves to quantification. This seems nicely, or eerily, to capture our approach to life in the contemporary phase of late capitalism extremely well, so I shall provide a brief reading of modern society through this slogan.

Doing more has become a goal in itself, for example, regardless of what one does. The Danish philosopher Anders Fogh Jensen (2009) has analyzed what he calls "the *project* society" and the corresponding social character of the "project *man*". These terms refer to the tendency of putting as many projects as possible into our lives. The main existential problem is no longer, as it was in the earlier society of prohibitions, that one wants too much and cannot conform to the rules (see also Bauman, 2007); rather, our problem in the project society is that we never manage to do enough, that we never quite catch up. So, like airlines, we tend to overbook our lives with projects, because we suffer from the anxiety of *missing out* on something. This means that our projects – in many arenas of our lives – become rather transitory and temporary, something we commit to only until something better shows up. This has been captured by another commercial slogan: *viz.* that of InterContinental Hotels: "You can't have a favorite place until you've seen them all". There is always a new place to see, a new job position to seek and a new partner to fall in love with. The ideal of the restless project or consumer society is "doing more", regardless of what one does. The downside is all sorts of problems with loyalty, commitment and long-term existential quests, as Richard Sennett argued so convincingly in the *Corrosion of Character* in the late 1990s (Sennett, 1998).

Today, many of us have calendars, to-do lists and applications for our smart phones that are meant to assist us in doing as much as possible. For psychiatric problems such as ADHD, there exist specific apps that are meant to help the patient monitor and measure everything from brushing her teeth in the morning to assessing her fitness for driving a car. ADHD Angel, for example, reminds the user when to take medicine and visit the doctor, and everything is framed within a quantitative logic of scales and self-assessments. These apps also exist for many other conditions, and over 100,000 medical and health apps have now been listed on the Apple App Store and Google Play (Lupton & Jutel, 2015). According to Lupton and Jutel, who have analyzed a large number of such apps, almost one third of American smart phone users (equivalent to 46 million people in the US alone) used these apps in January 2014. They represent a new way of being a patient – a "digitally engaged patient" (p. 129) – which involves a liberalization of the patient role. The patient often comes to the doctor's surgery not to receive a diagnosis, but to have the doctor validate the diagnosis that the patient has already decided on for herself.

Bowker and Star raise a warning flag in connection with the tendency to understand oneself through measurement technologies: "As we are socialized to become that which can be measured by our increasingly sophisticated measurement tools, the classifications increasingly naturalize across wider scope" (Bowker & Star, 2000, p. 326). And they continue on a pessimistic note: "we are taking a series of increasingly irreversible steps toward a given set of highly limited and problematic descriptions of what the world is and how we are in the world" (p. 326). To return to the analysis from Chapter 3, it means that our languages of suffering become narrowed down to the one favoured by a quantitative approach. The patient becomes not just a patient in the literal sense of simply passively receiving the diagnostic category (asking "what does the doctor tell me?"), but also an active consumer of health knowledge, including mental health categories and interventions, which, however, means that his or her afflictions are only addressed as health problems and disorders to be measured and not, for example, as social, moral or existential problems.

The numerous apps applied in self-diagnosis and tracking typically deal directly with measuring *how well* the user feels at a certain moment (and then systematically tracking the waxing and waning of how one feels over time), which takes us to the next element of the pharmaceutical slogan. "Feeling better" initially appears to be a goal that one cannot disagree with. Again, however, it easily lends itself to a purely quantitative interpretation, whereby one should feel as good *as possible*. More than anything else, this is today measured on various Likert scales, self-assessments, self-tracking devices and applications, not just for diagnosable conditions like depression, but also in relation to stress, for instance, using the stress test that many of us have on our smartphones as apps. Feeling better is a matter of degree, something that is always open for improvement. (Very different, say, from James Brown's "I feel good", which strikes one as more of an all or nothing exclamation.) If one takes antidepressants, one should as a matter of course continually monitor whether this makes one feel better (that is the whole point of it), and if one goes to the cognitive behavioural therapist, one is met by various score sheets to fill in week after week concerning how one feels. There is perhaps nothing intrinsically wrong with this, but it does invite one to see one's moods and emotions as something that can be detached from one's subjectivity "for control and clarification", as Eva Illouz says in her analysis of what she calls "emotional capitalism", involving not only what she calls a "textualization" of the subject (one's self-understanding being reduced to the linguistic categories available, for example on self-tracking apps), but certainly also a quantification (Illouz, 2007, p. 229).

Recently, Mikka Nielsen has interviewed adults diagnosed with ADHD and found examples of (in my words) people mediating their self-understanding through the textualizing and quantifying apps. Nielsen recalls one episode from her fieldwork, when she was interviewing 'Peter' about his ADHD:

> As a researcher, I am interested in ADHD as phenomenon and diagnostic category and I have acquainted myself with the theoretical literature on the diagnosis and its symptoms. But I am also interested in the phenomenological experience of living with ADHD. I want to get an insight into the experience of

> ADHD and optimistically try to get as close as possible to the immediate bodily experience and sensations of ADHD. I look into my interview guide and ask Peter how he experiences ADHD in his body and how ADHD affects him. Peter nods, looks down at his phone, finds a webpage about ADHD and reads aloud from the symptom descriptions. I listen to Peter's reading, but get impatient and annoyed that Peter is just reading from a web page and not explaining his experiences to me in his own words. (Nielsen, 2015, p. 13)

After the interview, Nielsen comes to the conclusion that "Peter's description of ADHD though the diagnostic descriptions is a part of how Peter experiences ADHD. He makes use of an available diagnostic vocabulary that concretely describes his experiences of ADHD and his bodily experience of ADHD and his understanding of ADHD as a diagnostic category are intermingled" (Nielsen, 2015, p. 14). This is a clear example of semiotic mediation and of the interrelatedness of diagnosis as a textual and quantifiable entity on the one hand, and the experience of being a certain way on the other.

Viewing oneself in a quantitative way normally means viewing oneself in terms of what one is *lacking* (more projects, better feelings, more focus etc.), which is something that becomes visible through the various quantitative measures. Axel Honneth (2008) refers to this as self-reification: we today consider our thoughts and emotions as discrete, measurable entities within us, like properties that can be owned and produced. In this sense, as Alastair Morgan has recently argued, "intimate life and emotions are turned into objects of calculation that can be captured quantitatively" (Morgan, 2014, pp. 228–229). The risk is that we ignore the worldly *import* of our emotions and feelings, so to speak; that is to say, we forget to concern ourselves with the *reasons* we have (or lack) for feeling certain ways. Want to feel better? Yes please! But no matter what? Probably not, and if our thoughts and feelings are world-directed, and can inform us of moral aspects of the world – which is a view of emotions that goes as far back as Aristotle – we can easily feel better for the wrong reasons. A purely quantitative approach simply accepts the mental objects as being *there*, something to observe and measure, and thus forgets the ways that they are entangled with what happens in the world. This parallels the critique of psychiatric diagnoses that they risk isolating the individual from the world and only take an interest in discrete symptoms "inside" the individual.

Living longer is the third goal in GlaxoSmithKline's triad. This is perhaps the one that most obviously belongs within a quantitative logic of life. Living longer has become a goal in itself, for many individuals and indeed for certain states (such as Denmark, where the former Prime Minister made it public policy that we should each live four-and-a-half years longer), seemingly without regard for the quality of the additional years that one lives, or the means that must be implemented in order to reach the goal of living longer. Again, there is nothing wrong with living longer as such, just as there is nothing wrong with doing more and feeling better, but it certainly seems to depend on *what* one does if one does more, *why* one feels better and *how* one lives. The purely quantitative logic that is at work in the slogan of GlaxoSmithKline is a very general logic in contemporary society that risks disregarding the values and qualitative distinctions between different *ways* of doing, feeling and living.

The Psychiatric Subject and its Quantified Self

A case can be made that it is this quantitative logic that is at work in contemporary diagnostic cultures in general. Notably, as we have seen, the contemporary diagnostic manuals are constructed around certain key assumptions about mental illness: *that* there is a boundary between the normal and the sick, *that* there are discrete mental illnesses, and *that* psychiatry's focus should primarily be on the biological aspects of mental illness (Angel, 2012, p. 8). In previous chapters, I have written about the revolution that took place in psychiatry around 1980 with the creation of DSM-III, which replaced the older etiological understanding of mental illness with a purely diagnostic understanding, based on actual symptoms within a given period of time (Horwitz, 2002). As we have seen, before DSM-III, a diagnosis was formulated on the background of the patient's biography and his or her experiences, actions and relationships, and psychiatrists often employed theoretical terminology when describing the patient, typically drawn from psychoanalysis. Unfortunately, this diagnostic practice was quite unreliable, which prompted the shift to the diagnostic approach of DSM-III and beyond, most recently DSM-5 (from May 2013). Now, a diagnosis is formulated if the patient has at least x number of symptoms from a given list within y weeks or months (depending on the specific diagnostic category). In other words, the diagnostic process has shifted to a quantitative logic of counting. A disorder is framed by counting symptoms and not primarily through a qualitative understanding of the person and her life problems within particular contexts and relationships.

The psychiatric vocabulary of the DSM in particular has travelled widely outside medical and psychiatric circles, and has become inscribed in people's everyday understandings of suffering and distress. As I have argued following Pickersgill, the DSM now operates as a "connective tissue" for many different groups with a stake in psychiatry (Pickersgill, 2012, p. 331). Armstrong (1995) has charted how medicine in general has developed historically into what he calls contemporary Surveillance Medicine, which functions by targeting everyone through screenings, surveys, a focus on risk factors, and a problematization of the normal. Everyone may now diagnose herself quantitatively by taking tests in magazines, self-help literature, or on the internet. Or we are diagnosed when taking part in some of the large-scale epidemiological studies that demonstrate that in any one year, more than a third of the European population could be diagnosed with a mental or brain disorder (Wittchen, Jacobi, & Rehm, 2011). Again, this is done through counting and quantification, and not through qualitative interpretations of people's life situations.

To sum up: psychiatric language and its diagnostic categories have become more important for our self-understanding than ever before. We use such terms to understand the behaviours, reactions and emotions of ourselves and others, and, by way of various looping-effects, as Hacking (1995b) has emphasized, we can become psychiatric subjects – and not just psychiatric subjects, but *diagnostic* psychiatric subjects. We become people that understand our problems and afflictions with reference to quantitative measures. The psychiatric subject emerges today as a quantified self – and often as a self-quantifiable self with willing patients subjecting themselves to this kind of logic. This is a result of a long historical process within the psy sciences, in particular psychology, as we shall now see.

From Quantitative Tools to Theories of the Subject: Ontologizing Processes

Human subjectivity is in many ways affected by the practices and discourses available in the given culture. This lies at the heart of Hacking's analyses of looping effects and is a premise of this book's investigation of how diagnostic cultures influence their cultural participants (and vice versa). There is one specific way that looping effects may occur, which has been described as a move "from tools to theories". This is particularly relevant if one wants to understand how quantitative measures come to influence the subjectivities they are meant to address.

In Danziger's classic work on the constitution of the psychological subject (Danziger, 1990) (which we also encountered in Chapter 2 on diagnoses as epistemic objects), he argued that a subject that was initially created under experimental conditions in psychological laboratories has since been exported to the rest of the world. This means that it was the very methods in psychology – experiments and tests – which led psychologists to devise new models of human beings, which again became part of the self-understanding of these human beings. Danziger has argued that the subjects studied by psychologists came to see themselves in terms of psychologists' research methods. Psychology's quantitative methods were "ontologized", to use a technical term; that is, read into the structure of the subject matter they were meant to investigate (see Brinkmann, 2011a, on which the following sections are based). In order to understand this, and understand how a similar process has more recently occurred with respect to psychiatric diagnostics, it might be useful to take a look at the quantitative test and how it developed historically.

Francis Galton was the main figure behind the institution of testing in Britain. In 1884 he charged every person who came to be tested ("measured") in his laboratory the sum of three pence, and more than 9,000 people showed up. However, as Danziger remarks, Galton's interest in devising his "antropometric measurement" was not financial, but in how the data could be useful in his eugenics programme (Danziger, 1990, p. 56). Galton was one of the leading architects of the "scientific racism" of the 19th century (Richards, 1996, p. 164) and he was very much interested in practical social planning. The Galtonian mental tests later became part of school life in the form of scientifically based examinations (p. 109) and they entered clinics, factories, and the military (Rose, 1999).

A main point emerging from Danziger's history of the subject in psychology is that from the very beginning of the 20th century, psychology became an applied science, and an extremely successful one, which became involved in the constitution of its subjects. Its applied aspects gradually led to a psychologization of society. Psychological practices did not spread because of a theoretical insight into what the mind is like; rather, it was its specific investigative methods that made everyone see herself or himself in psychology's image, leading to the ontologization of the quantitative methods.

This ontologization process frequently happens when psychology identifies its measures with the objects investigated. The categories of stimulus and response represent an instructive example (Danziger, 1996, p. 21). Stimulus and response are intelligible and common as units of measurement in psychology, but a lot of work has to be done by psychologists to crystallize such units in experimental practices. Neither our phenomenological experiences nor our stream of behaviour come neatly and discretely prefigured and arranged into these units. They are not "given" in nature to be picked up. Imagining and arranging human lives in terms of stimuli and responses demands a highly constricted experimental environment, but, as Danziger remarks, "stimuli and responses were always discussed as though they were features of the objective world and not artefacts of psychological procedure" (p. 21). These units, produced and employed by psychologists, were then identified with the "ultimate building blocks of reality" (p. 21), and when human beings begin to interpret their own and others' behaviour in light of what psychology tells them are the ultimate building blocks of psychological reality, we have come full circle in the process whereby methods are ontologized.

Modern investigations of mental life (psychology and psychiatry) began life with an object of investigation inherited from a certain cultural and philosophical tradition (Danziger, 1996), and from there, psychology went on:

> to apply certain procedures of experimentation and quantification to the study of the preexisting object. But once the disciplinary apparatus of investigation had been institutionalized, the possibility emerged of allowing this apparatus, rather than tradition, to define the objects of psychological science. (Danziger, 1996, p. 22)

Often the procedures came to dictate the theoretical formulations rather than the other way around (Danziger, 1996). The clearest example of psychology having identified its methods with its objects (ontologizing methods) is found in statistics, which also plays a huge role in current epidemiological programmes of screening and intervening, randomized controlled trials and many other medical and psychological practices. Statistics originally emerged, as its name testifies, as a "science of state" (Rose, 1996, p. 111), as a technology intended to gather information about states' populations in order to govern them. Hacking (1990) has argued that in the 19th century, with the development of statistical tools (largely due to psychologists such as Galton and Spearman), the belief spread that statistical laws expressed real laws inherent in social life. Statistical laws were no longer understood as simply expressing underlying deterministic events, for "statistical regularity underlay the apparently disorderly variability of phenomena" (Rose, 1996, p. 112). Statistics were ontologized: the world itself was seen as ordered statistically.

This has also been analyzed by Gerd Gigerenzer in an investigation of how psychological discoveries are dependent on psychologists' methods of providing justification for their knowledge claims (Gigerenzer, 1996). Gigerenzer's analysis demonstrates that "Scientists' tools for justification provide the metaphors and concepts for their theories" (p. 36) and that "Discovery is inspired by justification" (p. 46). In psychology, the role of statistical tools was very important in this regard: "After the institutionalization of inferential statistics, a broad range of cognitive processes, conscious and unconscious, elementary and complex, was reinterpreted as involving 'intuitive statistics'" (p. 39). Psychological theories of the mind were formulated with clear inspiration from the new methods and tools for data analysis, rather than from new data (p. 38). With the advent of statistics, the mind of the human being itself was being framed as a statistician.

Already in the 1940s, Egon Brunswik had claimed that people are intuitive statisticians (Smith, 1997, p. 838). Later on, the computer also became an extremely important tool that inspired widespread cognitive theories about the mind. Thereby, the algorithms and operations of the computer became ontologized. The view of humans as probabilistic rational choice machines – the *homo oeconomicus* – also owed much to the invention of statistics. Seen in this light, psychologists' methodological tools are not neutral, because the mind is continually recreated in their image (Gigerenzer, 1996, p. 55), and the statistical view in psychology has at times gained something approaching scientific hegemony. Danziger sums this up:

> The more rigidly the demands of a particular statistical methodology were enforced, the more effectively were ideas that did not fit the underlying model removed from serious consideration. Such ideas had first to be translated into a theoretical language that conformed to the reigning model before they could be seriously considered. In other words, they had to be eviscerated to the point where they no longer constituted a threat to the dominant system of preconceptions guiding investigative practices. The final stage of this process was reached when the statistical models on which psychologists had based their own practice were duplicated in their theories about human cognition in general. (Danziger, 1990, p. 155)

When it had become evident that the object of psychological research – the mind itself – works statistically, there was all the reason in the world to concentrate on this method when doing psychological science. Methods and theories then confirmed each other circularly. This is the from-tools-to-theories link, which comes full circle when taken up by subjects in processes of looping effects. As early as 1955, more than 80 per cent of published experimental articles in scientific journals used inferential statistics as a means of justification (Smith, 1997, p. 838). The experimental method of reasoning had, in the form of statistics, been introduced deeply into human subjects, who themselves were now portrayed as statisticians. This also contributed greatly to developing the image of human beings as creatures driven by causal powers rather than as agents capable of acting for meaningful moral reasons (which was the view of the mind articulated in Chapter 1 of this book). Rational choice machines can calculate the optimal way of reaching their goals, but they seem incapable of judging whether their goals are worth striving for. A mind described as a machine works mechanically and causally, but never normatively and morally.

This whole story is an example of how a quantitative image of human beings becomes a mirror of these human beings who begin to constitute themselves as such on macro cultural scales. It is a looping effect of human kinds, or macro ontologization of quantitative scientific methods. If it is true, as I have argued, that the psychiatric diagnostic vocabulary is becoming a very powerful language of suffering, then its quantitative and context-free (thus literally meaning-less) approach runs the risk of shaping human subjects in its image. The application – including the self-application of technologies (among them the numerous quantitative technologies) "changes what it is to be human", as Lock and Nguyen say (Lock & Nguyen, 2010, p. 23). The result might be a certain kind of self-fulfilling prophecy, whereby one's suffering is rendered meaningless because of the quantitative perspectives taken on it. This seems to fit perfectly with societal megatrends and their emphasis on the calculable, which some refer to as audit cultures (Strathern, 2000). Diagnostic cultures are deeply entangled with today's audit cultures in welfare societies, reducing suffering and all sorts of human problems to the calculable.

Diagnoses as Anchors in a Liquid World

Previously in this book I have tried to describe and analyze different functions that psychiatric diagnoses have in the lives of individuals. I will now suggest that in relation to society as a whole, diagnoses can be seen metaphorically as anchors that somehow promise to solidify people's experiences of suffering in a cultural situation that Bauman has described as liquid modernity (Bauman, 2007). Numbers and quantification seemingly add to the impression of solidity.

In today's liquid times, people's problems are rarely about "breaking free" from norms (that are experienced as liquid in the first place), but rather about "catching up" with developments that are experienced as constantly expanding. Perhaps this can be explained through an anecdote (recounted in Brinkmann, 2013b): I recently heard an experienced sexologist being interviewed on the radio, who said that people used to come to her clinic because they had too much desire and sexual drive, something they felt was problematic and possibly even pathological. Now, she told the listeners, this has changed, and people in general come to her clinic because they have too little sexual drive. Although this is just an anecdote, I believe it illustrates a fundamental change in our conception of human problems: wanting too much in a society of prohibitions is no longer people's main difficulty; rather, wanting too little in a society of excess is.

This is what Bauman has been trying to pinpoint in his writings on what he calls liquid modernity. Under such conditions, he believes, we witness a fundamental change in the sources of human suffering. Our problems and disorders used to originate from a profusion of prohibitions, but nowadays they tend to grow from an oversupply of possibilities. In plain terms, this means that the statement: "I have done something wrong" is replaced by "I cannot catch up" as a fundamental explanation of human distress. In Bauman's words, the consequence is:

> ...that depression arising from the terror of inadequacy will replace the neurosis caused by the horror of guilt (that is, of the charge of nonconformity that might follow a breach in the rules) as the most characteristic and widespread psychological affliction of the denizens of the society of consumers. (Bauman, 2007, p. 94)

We increasingly orient ourselves according to the antinomy of the possible and the impossible rather than the antinomy of the allowed and the forbidden. This does not mean that norms as such disappear and that "everything" is suddenly allowed. Rather, it means that some of our most important norms in society become oriented to performance and the future in a new way. "You have to!" becomes a more pervasive demand than "You may not!" One might say that it is no longer allowed not to do the possible, not to live up to one's "potentials", not to realize one's true self etc. (Petersen, 2011). Self-realization and human potential movements have become democratised, and are no longer the privilege of a small elite. Self-realization has become a duty; a demand of the masses that is centrally involved in the reproduction of late modern capitalist society (Honneth, 2004). Marginalization no longer follows from a transgression of the norms only, but – to put the matter paradoxically – from a failure to transgress, develop and constantly be on the move. As indicated by the sexology example above; the problem is no longer a surplus of desire, but a lack of it. In accordance with these transformations, we see that functional and even managerial languages are replacing moral languages when it comes to understanding human misery. Suffering is now rarely seen as a meaningful moral reaction to events, but becomes a mental dysfunction; a sign that one has not lived up to the demands of change, flexibility and constant desire. As many social analysts of the current "age of depression" have argued, a lack of desire is a key symptom of illness in a culture that valorizes development and self-realization above all else (Petersen, 2011). In a "society of consumers" (Bauman,

2007), one is easily seen as suffering from some pathology or other, if one does not have the desire or will to consume, develop and engage in lifelong learning.

Humans have always experienced various kinds of suffering, and they have always sought to understand their suffering through some kind of meaning system. This was what I tried to analyse in Chapter 2 with the notion of "languages of suffering". But when meaning systems are liquefied, along with the transformation of society into liquid modernity, humans begin to look for new ways of anchoring their experiences of suffering, which I suggest happens now by way of reference to the diagnostic system and the different attempts to quantify suffering through diagnostic tests, apps and self-help literature. This was what prompted the shift to DSM-III in 1980: a wish to create a more reliable and solid system that was not dependent on the different qualitative assessments of the diagnosticians. However, as I have also tried to show, individuals who are diagnosed have a tendency to take on the identity offered by the diagnostic system, which, in its new guises, mean a quantified system. This leads to quantifiable selves in processes of looping effects.

This happens not just on the individual level, when persons are diagnosed by general practitioners or psychiatrists with reference to numerical tests or are monitoring their mental health by using smart phone apps. As Nielsen and Grøn have demonstrated, it also happens collectively or on institutional levels in health education programmes (Nielsen & Grøn, 2013). Nielsen and Grøn have conducted ethnographic fieldwork in six different health education programmes, which are within the somatic fields, but the focus on the use of numbers and self-assessment warrants some generalization to psychiatry. It appears from the fieldwork that "not only health professionals, but also lay persons incorporate [a] quantitative understanding of the body when they use different devices to measure and keep track of their health" (p. 62). Participation in the patient schools is based on numbers (in a diagnostic sense), and the use of scales in particular becomes a way of "assessing, paying attention to, and giving voice to bodily sensations" (p. 66). In this way, subjective experience and biomedical knowledge become linked, albeit in a way that also affects people's sense of themselves: "The use of scales offers a language and can be understood as an attempt to capture an uncanny field between numbers and experience, between biomedicine and phenomenology, between the objective and subjective body" (p. 67). So numbers are used as inscription devices that are not only *means* through which individuals may know themselves, but they are also *mediators* that transform what they are concerned with. They become inscribed on a subject, who is an active participant in this kind of self-inscription, but they are at the same time involved in creating a quantified identity, which is a primary practice through which psychiatric subjectivity is created in the 21st century.

A Self of Qualitative Distinctions

If this is a valid analysis, should it be a cause for alarm? What is wrong with being subjectified as a quantified self? The answer given by Charles Taylor and others, which I find utterly persuasive, is that something crucial about human subjectivity is lost if we overlook the qualitative dimensions of existence and interpret our afflictions in purely quantitative terms. When writing about the crisis in the European sciences, Edmund Husserl, the founder of phenomenology, put it like this, with an early sensitivity to what Hacking would decades later refer to as the looping effects of human kinds: "purely factual sciences make purely factual men" (Husserl, 1954) – and women, we should add. Quantities and facts are related, just as qualities and values are, so if we simplify, we can say that a purely factual psychiatry makes purely quantitative subjects.

Charles Taylor's argument, at least since the early 1980s and culminating in *Sources of the Self* (1989), is that our identity, our sense of who we are, is inextricably "linked to the stand we take on issues of concern, and for that we need points of orientation, the reference points provided by frameworks of *qualitative* contrast", to quote his exegete, Nicholas Smith (Smith, 2002, p. 97; my italics). Such frameworks are given us to discover and articulate rather than something to freely choose. These frameworks are based on traditions and communities, on shared practices, institutions, and the social imaginary, and not on personal choice or private self-reflection. According to Taylor, we presuppose frameworks of qualitative contrasts in our everyday lives when we explain ourselves to others. When we give accounts of our actions, we offer descriptions and justifications in the light of our motives in the situation and try to show that the situation justifies our acting in a certain way. Sometimes we explain ourselves in light of our desires and preferences (asking ourselves: "what do I want the most?"), which is what Taylor (1985) calls weak evaluation, where we simply weigh our desires and determine which is quantitatively the *strongest*. But if the quantitative model of weak evaluation were the only model a person had recourse to in deliberating and explaining herself, we would find that this person led an extremely impoverished and inhuman life. All she could do would be to act on her strongest desire at any given moment. Such a person could never articulate a genuine reason for her actions, for she could not refer to any moral frameworks; all she could say would be that she did something because her strongest desire made her do so. In that sense, she could only refer to causes and not to reasons. If acting means acting for a reason, such an individual could not act at all. She would be an utterly "quantified self", pushed by the strongest force, but incapable of acting for a reason.

Central to Taylor's theory of agency is the observation that as persons, we not only have desires, but also second-order desires (that is, desires about which desires to have). We have the capacity for evaluating our desires, but in light of what? If we could only evaluate desires in the light of other desires, we would be caught in the quantitative logic, and it would merely be a matter of determining which desire were strongest. Then we could never have a reason to change our desires, and this runs counter to our everyday moral experience where we are in fact often concerned with changing our desires for moral reasons, and not just because other desires are quantitatively stronger. Taylor here introduces his famous notion of strong evaluation. Strong evaluation is "when the goods putatively identified are not seen as constituted as good by the fact that we desire them, but rather are seen as normative for desire" (Taylor, 1981, p. 193). In strong evaluation we are concerned with the *qualitative* worth of our motivations, desires and ways of life. Is what we want desir*able*? The strength of our desires does not matter here; rather, the issue is whether what we desire is worth desiring. Taylor's point is that we simply cannot do without a qualitative vocabulary that refers to the moral frameworks within which we live our lives – if we want to be *bona fide* agents with some kind of identity (Taylor, 1989). In relation to diagnostic cultures, his argument can be said to imply that we cannot fully understand human suffering in abstraction from a qualitative vocabulary and moral frameworks. Without these, suffering collapses into meaningless entities that can be measured and counted (as in diagnostic systems), but without reference to the worldly contexts in which people suffer. Taylor's idea of strong evaluation represents a version of what cultural psychologists call semiotic mediation (Valsiner, 2007): a process through which persons create distance from their preferences and tendencies in the here and now by way of signs and symbols in order to act, with the goal of evaluating these preferences and tendencies in light of values, including moral values. As human persons, we are creatures who not only relate to the world as other animals also do, but who are also capable of relating to *how* we relate to the world, which was also Kierkegaard's famous definition of a self, brought forth in *The Sickness unto Death* (Kierkegaard, 1849).

Much more can be said about Taylor's theory of the self as navigating within a moral space of qualitative distinctions, orienting itself in terms of what is always already important (see Brinkmann, 2008). Here, however, the point is simply to articulate the contrast between the idea that the self or our identity is defined by such qualitative (and moral) commitments and the diagnostic idea of a quantified self. GlaxoSmithKline's slogan is merely a radicalization of the quantified self that aims to do more, feel better and live longer, regardless of the qualitative worth of doing so.

The charge against currents diagnostics – that diagnoses such as depression and anxiety lead to a collapse of the distinction between normal human suffering and mental disorder – can be related to the discussion of the quantified self, for if mental disorder is approached in purely quantitative terms, literally by counting symptoms, then it becomes difficult, sometimes impossible, to distinguish between, say, a person's agonizing feeling of guilt after having done something wrong (which may lead to "symptoms" such as weight loss, sleep disturbance and negative automatic thoughts about oneself) and clinical depression: if there are enough symptoms, then the condition counts as depression. That someone suffers from guilt can only be recognized through understanding the qualitative meanings of the person in a situation. This, of course, can be a very significant existential problem in a person's life, but this is not the same as saying that it is a mental disorder. Einstein allegedly said that it is not everything that can be counted that counts – and it is not everything that counts that can be counted. The quantitative approach to the subject and her life, institutionalized in many parts of psychiatry and the welfare state and mediated by numerous quantitative technologies, may lead us to disregard those important aspects of human suffering that cannot be counted, or to misinterpret them when we begin counting, resulting, for example, in diagnosing a case of existential guilt as clinical depression. Counting, quantifying, has many virtues, but can appear as an almost obsessive-compulsive social pathology in itself that may, sadly, create purely factual men and women.

Conclusions

Based on a historical account of the emergence of quantitative investigative practices in psychology and related disciplines, I have argued in this chapter that human beings have increasingly come to understand themselves in light of quantitative measures. We relate to ourselves more and more in quantitative terms, and this is something, I argued, that we also find on a macro sociological plane with the rise of audit cultures and the "do more, feel better, live longer" mentality incarnated in the slogan of GlaxoSmithKline. Our diagnostic cultures are today infused with quantification technologies, which are not neutral means of self-knowledge and regulation, but which mediate and co-constitute the subjects that they measure. Bauman has analyzed contemporary macro culture as liquid modernity, and, given these cultural conditions, it becomes understandable that people look for anchors that can at least temporarily stabilize their experiences of suffering and uncertainty, and psychiatric diagnoses appear to them as such anchors. However, the price seems to be that the quantitative logic that follows makes it difficult to understand the contextual and relational features that render suffering meaningful. Purely factual science may make purely factual men and women, as Husserl said, and purely quantitative diagnostics may make purely quantitative subjects.

Chapter 6

Interpreting the Epidemics

In this chapter I wish to present and discuss some of the most influential interpretations of the current "epidemics" of mental disorders. I put "epidemics" in quotation marks, because a key point of this book is that it is uncertain whether the rising number of people diagnosed represents a genuine growth in psychiatric problems or rather a pathologization of various ordinary human life problems. Have more people become ill because of modern society? Or have we always had these kinds of numbers of ill people among us, but are only now able to find them because of scientific advances? Are the disorders fabricated by *Big Pharma*? I argue that such interpretations may be legitimate in certain cases, but that two others are more significant: one that is concerned with the cultural-historical "psychiatrization" of suffering, and another that puts emphasis on changed diagnostic practices. After reviewing these interpretations, I turn directly to the concept of pathologization and show how it comes in many forms today (for example as self-pathologization, but also as stigmatization), and I argue that "the pathologization of everything" is a huge problem for a number of reasons: it skews the resources available for treatment, it paradoxically leads to increased vulnerability of individuals, it routinely individualizes social problems (thereby leading to individualized "solutions", such as pills or therapy) and it narrows our self-understanding. In order to inform the discussion about the reasons for the rising number of people diagnosed, we need to understand the nature of mental disorders and psychiatric pathologies. What are these if looked at from cultural psychological perspectives? This question is taken up in the next chapter.

Mental Disorders Today: Epidemics or Pathologization?

As we have seen throughout this book, we live in a time and place where a psychiatric language and its diagnostic categories have become more important for our self-understanding than ever before. As I argued in Chapter 3, the diagnostic vocabulary has become our preferred "language of suffering" in many instances. The diagnoses are used as semiotic mediators for a huge number of purposes, and words with specific meanings within the discipline of psychiatry, such as stress, anxiety, depression and mania, have become part of our everyday vocabularies. We can refer to this as *diagnostic expansion*, a process involving the emergence of various diagnostic cultures, in which people use the diagnostic terms for many different reasons and within many different kinds of social practice. But the diagnostic expansion is broader than this. It operates in (at least) three stages.

First, more people are in fact diagnosed with psychiatric problems than before. Of course, there are some diagnoses that remain outside this development, but for many non-psychotic diagnoses such as depression, anxiety and ADHD, we are seeing a significant rise in contemporary times. Second, many epidemiologists will claim that far more people *ought* to be diagnosed than is actually the case. There is a huge *treatment gap*, as it is called, which often indicates that only around half of the people (or even fewer) who should be diagnosed (because they have the symptoms) are in fact diagnosed (Kohn, Saxena, Levav & Saraceno, 2004). Thus, people are ill without being discovered, which – from a health perspective – is quite a scandal. Imagine a similar finding in somatic medicine, in relation to cancer, for example, where it would undoubtedly be a cause for uproar.

Third, as many critics have argued more generally, there is an ongoing cultural process of pathologization, which means that many traits and behaviours that used to be considered normal human problems (sorrow, melancholia, guilt, shyness etc.) are now conceptualized as mental disorders that can be diagnosed and treated medically and therapeutically. This is also a fundamental assumption in this book, and we have previously seen how epidemiological studies demonstrate that more than a quarter of all men and women in the European Union, for example, will have symptoms of at least one psychiatric disorder in the course of just one year (Wittchen & Jacobi, 2005). This *may* be interpreted as representing genuine epidemics of depression, anxiety, social phobia etc., but, on an alternative and less dramatic interpretation (although perhaps rather more realistically), it may testify to a massive pathologization of human life; a breakdown of our conventional distinctions between problems in living and psychiatric disorders. A problem, according to the critics, is not just that so many parties – from the biomedical industry to psychotherapists – benefit from educating individuals in the art of interpreting their problems in light of medicine and psychology (Kutchins & Kirk, 1997), but also that such pathologization may make all of us more vulnerable when we employ the diagnostic language of suffering for evermore purposes, which invites everyone to see him or herself as a victim or patient.

Rose (2006) has tried to account for the diagnostic expansion with reference to five different hypotheses: (1) there is actually more mental disorder today than in previous times; (2) we are simply better at recognizing the various kinds of mental disorder that have always been there; (3) psychiatrists act as entrepreneurs that campaign for psychiatric expansion; (4) the pharmaceutical industry is chiefly responsible for distorting our perception and treatment of mental disorder; (5) there has been an overall cultural psychiatrization of human discontents.

Some of these hypotheses are partly overlapping and others are contradictory. With inspiration from this list, I shall try below to develop the hypotheses into viable interpretations, but I believe that numbers (3) and (5) on Rose's list are actually aspects of one process, so for that reason I have grouped them together. In addition, I have created a new fifth category, which pinpoints how diagnostic psychiatry changed at the end of the 20th century, which I believe to be so important that it deserves an explanatory or interpretative category of its own.

I should say that I believe that all of the interpretations are legitimate, as they are actually concerned with different aspects of our diagnostic cultures. Together they provide us with a near complete picture, but, if we imagine the diagnostic expansion as a jigsaw puzzle, we can perhaps say that not all interpretations give us an equal number of pieces of the puzzle.

The Societal Interpretation: There Are More Mentally Ill People Than Before

The first interpretation follows up on the previous chapter and its analyses of modernity, such as Zygmunt Bauman's, which emphasize the fluid, accelerating and uncertain nature of existence today. An entire industry of cultural analysis has depicted "the malaise of modernity", as Charles Taylor once put it (Taylor, 1991), demonstrating how humans suffer because of the effects of capitalism, urbanization, secularization and atomization. This cultural critique is as old as sociology and the social sciences themselves. Recently, cultural critics have often pointed to the effects of neo-liberalism, a form of governmentality whereby the individual is made responsible for numerous things in his or her life, including, perhaps, distress and suffering. Others have argued that we have developed a fast-paced society that is constantly accelerating (Rosa, 2003). In this society, people have to engage in life-long learning and incessant self-optimization and self-realization, which has taken a form that Axel Honneth has called "organized self-realization" (Honneth, 2004). This is when self-realization no longer represents a struggle against the system (capitalism, the patriarchy etc.), which was the situation around the events of 1968, but instead has been transformed into an ideology that functions to render the system legitimate. In what Bauman calls *solid* modernity (which others refer to as industrial society), norms of living were organized around sets of prohibitions ("you must not do this or that!"). A struggle against the system thus involved a struggle to transgress the prohibitions. The subsequent phase of *liquid* modernity is instead organized around sets of demands ("you *should* do this and that!"). This means that people no longer develop problems when they come to *break* with the norms, but rather when they fail to *live up to* the demands of flexibility and change.

The modern competitive states in a globalized consumer economy are dependent on fluid and flexible individuals being constantly on the move. The sociological analysis of the effects of this cultural transformation, however, often looks at the downside and concludes, for example, that the rising numbers of people with depression results from chronic feelings of stress and a pressure to develop and realize oneself (Petersen, 2011). Depression, on this account, is a pathology of insufficiency, and societies in which people are never allowed to stand still might represent obstacles to healthy, sustainable lives. On a related note, Baroncelli (2015) has argued in a recent analysis that the order of meaning has changed in Western societies, notably pushed by neo-liberalism and the erection of money (and instrumentalism more generally) as a God. This ultimately leads to meaninglessness, making everyone vulnerable to depression, since this condition is characterized by emptiness and loss of meaning. As Rønberg (2014) has argued in her ethnographic study of depression, the people diagnosed often express a "no future" attitude of meaninglessness, as in the following quote from one of her informants: "I cannot imagine the future. I don't have any pictures of me sitting with a family. I have no pictures coming up in my head when I think about the future. It's all just black and white. I have no compass to navigate with anymore. I always used to have that. I'm tired now. It's not because I'm afraid of dying or something like that – but the future! (Michael, 38)" (p. 1). According to the societal interpretation of the diagnostic expansion, Michael is likely a victim of late-modern accelerated life and its loss of meaning, and his inability to form images of his future life is a major deficit in a culture that valorizes development and a forward-looking attitude.

Although this societal interpretation resonates with many, it is difficult to assess its scope and validity. On the one hand, it seems valid to conclude that society has undergone considerable fundamental transformations in the last 50 to 100 years, as scores of historians and sociologists have pointed out. It also seems probable that these transformations, and not least their pace, have made some people more vulnerable and receptive to various forms of psychopathology, but still, I do not think that this first interpretation can stand alone, and it does come with a number of problems. First, there is the problem of timeframe: it might be true that looking at the last few decades gives one the impression that more and more people are suffering from stress-related disorders, depression, anxiety and ADHD. However, what happens if we expand the viewpoint and go back, say, 100, 200 or even 500 years? Then it becomes increasingly impossible to say whether more or fewer people suffered from mental disorder. In any case, unless one is a staunch cultural pessimist, it seems fair to conclude that life has improved considerably for most people in many different ways, at least in the West, over the last 100 years, and very few of us (including most of the cultural critics) would want to return to the living conditions that were common before the First World War, for example.

The main problem with this first interpretation stems from the fact that we simply do not know how many people would qualify as mentally disordered if we were to go back more than just a few decades. Different psychiatric categories existed back then, different diagnostic tests (if any) and different treatments and there are actually some studies, of depression, for example, that seemingly demonstrate that there has not been a rise in prevalence. Murphy and colleagues (2000) compared studies from 1952, 1970 and 1992 and could not find an increase in the prevalence of depression. It is very difficult to assess whether depression and other such conditions are becoming more widespread or not, and this is something that calls for reservations about the first interpretation. Horwitz and Wakefield have even argued that anthropologists and critical sociologists, who are worried about the transformation of society, "have functioned as 'enablers' of psychiatry's over inclusive definitions of disorder" (2007, p. 194). A fair verdict might be that there probably is something about the ways that society now functions that causes new forms of suffering, but that it is quite speculative to conclude that these forms of suffering are best accounted for by using a psychiatric-diagnostic vocabulary. New experiences of distress may appear as part of a phenomenology of "not being able to catch up", but it is an open question whether these experiences represent psychopathological conditions.

The Official Interpretation: We Have Become Better at Finding the Ill

The next interpretation is in many ways complementary to the first, and it suffers from the same problems, albeit in almost precisely the opposite way. I refer to it as the "official interpretation", because it is one that many proponents of psychiatry would like to advance. We often hear, especially with regard to recent diagnoses like ADHD (which acquired this name only in 1987) that there have always been children (and likely also adults) who have suffered from this condition, but without anyone knowing it, because the category did not exist and no treatments or tests were available. If it was problematic to claim that there are more people suffering now (because we do not know how many people suffered from mental disorders just a few decades ago), it is equally problematic to claim that they have always been there but without anyone knowing it. So why do psychiatrists routinely tell this story? The obvious answer is that it portrays their discipline, which has otherwise failed to make progress comparable to what has been happening in somatic medicine, as a genuine cumulative science. Underpinning the "official interpretation", however, is the idea that like physics or chemistry (or physiology, to point to a discipline closer to psychiatry), new knowledge is constantly added to the knowledge base, which means that the discipline deserves recognition, funding and everything that follows from that.

Like the first interpretation, this interpretation is somewhat speculative due to the lack of reliable data from the past, and it furthermore builds on a questionable premise: that "mental disorders simply await their recognition by adequate diagnostic schemes", as Rose has put it (Rose, 2006, p. 475). This is a species of strong essentialism positing that symptoms and disorders are everywhere the same and that only our conceptual characterizations vary across time and place. As I try to show in this book (most directly in the next chapter), there is a much more convincing story to tell about mental disorder if one admits that such phenomena are constituted by many different forces and actors, some of which are related to the person's body and brain, while others are related to social practices and discursive categories. In my view, we should beware of all-encompassing and simplistic accounts, so while it seems plausible to say that a serious mental problem such as schizophrenia – with relatively well-defined symptoms – is likely a relatively stable entity, which was also problematic for people before it was named as such, we should at the same time remain open to the view that other disorders are of a different kind and might be constituted – in part or even in their entirety – by the categories we apply to them. This is what Hacking has described as "making up people" (Hacking, 1986), which I referred to in Chapter 2.

We may conclude about this second interpretation that it might work for certain (probably very few) disorders such as schizophrenia, but for the majority of disorders, we are dealing with phenomena that are much more responsive to cultural forces and social practices, and which do not have an unchanging essence across time and place that we have finally come to frame precisely with our current diagnostic vocabulary. The second interpretation also has the more immediate problem that many of today's diagnoses and tests seem "over inclusive" (Wakefield, 2010), which means that psychiatrists may not simply finally have found the people that have always been disordered, but rather are putting forward the false claim that many people with common human problems are suffering from a mental illness or disorder.

The Critical Interpretation: Towards Pharmageddon?

This leads us to the next and more critical interpretations. The third looks at the role of psychopharmacology. There are (at least) two ways that the medical industry can be said to be co-responsible for the diagnostic expansion. I mentioned the first one above: the industry has an interest not only in selling drugs to help alleviate people's symptoms, but also in "selling sickness" (Moynihan & Cassels, 2005). If the industry succeeds in convincing doctors and patients that something is a disorder for which they have a remedy, then a market appears where the companies can sell their drugs. In the US, companies are now allowed to engage in Direct to Consumer Advertising (which was made legal in 1997, New Zealand being the only other country in the world where this is permitted), where the adverts often end with the message "Ask your doctor!", whenever the troubled person can recognize the advertised "symptoms". So, the industry is a powerful agent in pathologization processes, not just in the West, but on a global scale, as Ethan Watters has recently documented in his book on the globalization of the American psyche (Watters, 2010). Depression in the Western sense (which can allegedly by targeted by drugs) came to Japan only in the 1990s, for example, because there was a huge market that had not yet been exploited. This represents a threat not only to people's rights not to be pathologized, but also to culturally engrained "folk psychiatries" that die out or are Americanized.

The other way that psychopharmacology is involved in the expansion of diagnoses is even more serious, and this takes us to the concept of 'Pharmageddon', recently articulated by David Healy (2012). The point here is that drugs have severe iatrogenic effects that in more than a few cases actually make people more ill than they would have been without the drugs. Healy states that a quarter of all deaths in hospitals are due to effects of pharmaceuticals, and it is becoming more and more obvious that many drugs against psychiatric symptoms are quite dangerous. Some critics of the industry argue that drugs might be needed in the most severe cases of mental disorder, when we talk about the worst forms of depression, for example, but in less severe cases, it might be difficult to justify the widespread use of drugs such as antidepressants. In about half of the studies that have been conducted, antidepressants do *not* come out as better than placebo (p. 77), and it is estimated that only around ten per cent of the patients treated respond specifically to the antidepressants (p. 83). Thus, very large numbers of people in the Western world take antidepressants (for example, in Denmark, around eight per cent of the population consume antidepressants daily), yet in many cases it is overwhelmingly likely that the only effects of the drugs are placebo and side-effects. Thus, the lives of these people might actually become worse because of the drugs, and this also explains why around half of the patients who begin a treatment with antidepressants stop before the treatment programme has come to an end: the side-effects are experienced as worse than the disorder.

It thus seems that what is needed is a sociological explanation of the success of Big Pharma, when the actual medical success is quite limited, at least for some of the commonly prescribed drugs. Healy shows that the marketing budgets for the large players in the industry are larger than their budgets for research and development of new drugs. In a consumer society, the medical industry is a powerful agent in selling (promises of) health and well-being. On a similar note, in his best-selling critique of the pharmaceutical industry, Whitaker (2010) asks the fundamental and very interesting question: how can it be that since the mid-1950s, when the first psychopharmacological drugs were invented, the number of people who suffer from a mental disorder has seemingly just gone up? One would have expected the opposite development: when new medical interventions are used, the number of symptoms and problems should go down. The proponents of the drugs like to point out how successful they have been in treating mental disorder, and this leads Whitaker to observe:

> Given this great advance in care, we should expect that the number of disabled mentally ill in the United States, on a per-capita basis, would have declined over the past fifty years. [...] Instead, as the psychopharmacology revolution has unfolded, the number of disabled mentally ill in the United States has *skyrocketed*. (Whitaker, 2010, p. 5)

In the rest of his award-winning book, Whitaker articulates his own, quite disturbing, answer to this paradox: through readings of major studies of long-term effects of psychiatric drugs, he argues that the reason lies in the pills themselves. They actually make people's lives worse. As Whitaker concludes: "In large part, this epidemic [of the number of disabled mentally ill] is iatrogenic in kind" (Whitaker, 2010, p. 208). Thus, it is the result of the workings of doctors, in particular those representing the psy-disciplines (notably psychopharmacology). The concept of iatrogenesis goes back to Ivan Illich in the 1970s, and his analyses have since been corroborated to the extent that there is now "incontrovertible epidemiological evidence that prescription drugs are a common cause of illness and death" (Lock & Nguyen, 2010, p. 70).

This is quite a dramatic conclusion, which – on the one hand – looks convincing because of the scores of studies, including Cochrane reviews, which can be mobilized to support it. But, on the other hand, it is also likely true that many people's lives have been saved because of the drugs that they have taken to alleviate various psychiatric symptoms. Both doctors and patients report this, and from my fieldwork with people diagnosed with ADHD, I have been told many times by people who are using the drugs, that the medication has changed their lives for the better. So the issue seems to be a standard one in the medical sciences, involving a clash between a logic of evidence (which often, but not always, counts against the use of drugs) and a logic of personal experience (where many people, but not everyone, benefits from using the drugs). As with all forms of medicine, the pills work differently in different organisms, so perhaps it is no surprise that people react differently to the psychiatric drugs they are using. Perhaps the solution is more "personalized medicine", or perhaps psychiatry should return to studying how to improve the lives of the suffering through social and contextual means, rather than focusing overwhelmingly on psychopharmacology (even if this will not always cure the disordered)?

In any case, it seems fair to say that the jury is still out, debating the role of *Big Pharma* in creating (and alleviating) suffering in modern times. What is clear, however, is that the possibility of a rational discussion of these issues would be much improved if the pharmaceutical industry lost some of its power over testing and marketing new drugs. The "filer drawer problem", for example, is well-known: the problem of negative results of drug trials not being published, because the research is paid for by the companies. Knowing how many people – children, adolescents, adults, and old people – who are in fact treated with psychopharmacological medicine in our diagnostic cultures ought to lead to increased control over the workings of the medical industry. In conclusion we may reasonably state that the *Big Pharma* interpretation does provide us with some pieces to the jigsaw puzzle, but that there are certainly also other factors at work. This follows (among other reasons) from the simple fact that many of the psychiatric conditions that are seemingly growing today (such as personality disorders) are *not* treated with drugs, which means that the effect of the industry is at most indirect in these cases.

The Cultural-historical Interpretation: A Psychiatrization of the Human Condition

The next interpretation is the one that the present book primarily focuses on articulating in different ways. Its premise is that human suffering and eccentricity have somehow to be comprehended – by collectives, but certainly also by those who suffer – in the sense that experienced problems and distress have to be given some form or other. It is painful for human beings to suffer, but it is even more painful if one's suffering cannot be rendered meaningful, so people look for the interpretative resources that are available to ascribe some kind of meaning to the experienced problems and distress. In Chapter 3, I conceptualized these interpretative resources as "languages of suffering", and I subsequently approached them as "semiotic mediators" that people use to understand and cope with their problems. The *leitmotif* of this book has been to develop the argument that many different interpretative resources have been weakened or have even disappeared entirely in contemporary times: I have pointed to the eclipse of religious, existential, moral and political understandings of suffering that used to play a much larger role, while at the same time, the psychiatric-diagnostic vocabulary and its related set of practices have expanded enormously. Today, it seems fair to conclude that this conceptualization is the dominant one and is even, in some instances, hegemonic, thereby segregating other forms of understanding of pain and distress.

Thus, the cultural-historical development of modern societies has gone hand in hand with a psychiatrization of suffering specifically, and of the human condition more broadly. In this book I have approached this phenomenon from a cultural psychological perspective, looking at how people may come to *have*, *be*, and *do* their sufferings in ways that are informed by psychiatric diagnoses and the social practices in which these diagnoses make sense. Others have conceived of the phenomenon in Foucauldian terms, whereby psychiatry is comprehended as a technology of the self (Lock & Nguyen, 2010, p. 301). Psychiatry and its categories do not simply operate on a pre-cultural, authentic self, but are involved in the very constitution of the (suffering) self as such, a process Foucault would have called subjectification (Foucault, 1988; 1994). On both interpretations – the cultural psychological and the Foucauldian – the person is seen as an active participant in his or her self-formation; not, of course, as the only relevant agent, but as someone who is not simply a passive victim of whatever forces (social, discursive etc.) that happen to exist. Just as 'culture' – including what I call 'diagnostic cultures' in this book – is not a causal variable that affects the person from the outside, according to cultural psychologists, so power was not for Foucault some causal force that simply strikes the subject from the outside. Power, knowledge, freedom and ethics are famously connected from Foucault's perspective (where there is power, there is also freedom, for example, for otherwise it would be pure determinism), so this in fact brings his approach close to the cultural psychological one.

Together with Peter Musaeus, I have tried to show how a cultural psychological perspective can be combined with a Foucauldian take on technologies of the self (Musaeus & Brinkmann, 2011). Our study concerned family therapy and how a family appropriates semiotic resources from their therapy sessions and employs them in their daily life. We found through qualitative interviews (conducted in families' homes by Peter Musaeus) that family members incorporated a therapeutic language and signs from the therapy into their everyday regulation of action and emotions (for example, they had learned to say "STOP" loudly in order to halt an escalating conflict, and this they did during the interview in a way that hardly contributed to de-escalating the conflict). Thus, there was a semiosis (a sign process) that operated as a technology of the self to constitute the family dynamics, and all of it made sense within a framework set up by what Rose calls *psy*, which includes psychiatry and psychology (Rose, 1999). This is an example of how members of a family come to understand their lives and problems in light of psychiatric and psychological ideas and practices – and are active participants in this process.

All in all, this fourth interpretation focuses on the broad line of development through which modern societies have been psychiatrized. A large number of human problems are now approached through a diagnostic lens, many afflictions are reframed as mental disorders, and a system of treatment can be mobilized to intervene in the lives of children and adults when some problem is registered. Since this cultural-historical interpretation is rather sweeping, it is difficult to assess its precise scope and count exactly how many pieces it contributes to the jigsaw puzzle of diagnostic expansion. It is perhaps best approached as a kind of meta-narrative within which there is room for many other interpretations. One can say, for example, that it is likely that the psychiatrization of life that makes new discoveries of mental disorder possible (the second interpretation), and it is also what legitimates the widespread use of psychiatric drugs (the third interpretation). This interpretation may also be seen in conjunction with the last one I shall mention, which emphasizes the ways in which the technicalities of diagnostic practices have changed, which in itself contributes enormously to diagnostic expansion.

The Undeniable Interpretation: Changed Diagnostic Practices

The fifth and final interpretation of the expanding diagnostics has also already been touched upon several times in this book. It focuses on the ways that diagnostic practices have changed, particularly with the introduction of DSM-III in 1980. Since this is an undeniable historical fact, I refer to it (tongue in cheek) as the undeniable interpretation. Before DSM-III, a psychiatrist would suggest a diagnosis based on the patient's life story and experiences, often with a focus on childhood, since this was the heyday of psychoanalysis. The change from this etiological approach to diagnosis and to modern diagnostic psychiatry has been analyzed in a large number of publications, for example, by Horwitz (2002), as mentioned above. The change was prompted primarily by the unreliability of etiological diagnostics, which caused dissatisfaction among insurance companies in the US and also in welfare societies that are dependent on a reliable form of classification of people with mental disorders. The new diagnostic practice that was developed was based on current symptoms, rather than on patient history, and, today, the reigning logic states that someone has a mental illness or disorder if the person has at least x number of symptoms within y weeks or months (depending on the specific diagnostic category). Biographical depth is replaced by symptomatic breadth in the diagnostic process.

As we have seen, this provides for a more reliable diagnostic process, but it is likely at the expense of its validity, because the new system makes it immensely difficult to separate symptoms of mental disorder from unpleasant life phenomena. However, one can object that in many cases, the result of a symptom checklist is not allowed to stand alone. It figures as only one part of a diagnostic process, alongside a more thorough diagnostic interview, for example. This is true in many cases, and most doctors know that their situated judgment is very important in addition to the standardized tests. Nevertheless, there is a pressure toward standardization and manualization in modern health care. Increasingly, the experience and judgment of professionals is downplayed and instead, "evidence-based" knowledge, often legitimating the symptom checklists, is referred to as authoritative. Furthermore, most of the prevalence studies of mental disorder, including many cited in this book, are based on symptoms, which can be counted by using simple questionnaires. The result is often quite likely to be inflated rates of various mental problems, and the problem is that these rates are published not just in specialized professional journals (where the readers know that they should be taken with a grain of salt), but also in popular media, and are consumed by people in diagnostic cultures who are eager to read about the problems they might have. Thus, we come full circle in a kind of macroscopic looping effect (*pace* Hacking), where "panic statistics" about mental illness result in people interpreting their problems as instances of the various kinds of psychopathology, thus contributing to the rising numbers.

With these five interpretations of the current diagnostic expansion, I believe we have enough pieces of the jigsaw puzzle to see a general picture appearing. I believe the most trustworthy account of this phenomenon is one that argues that on the one hand, there have been developments in the knowledge base of psychiatry (second interpretation above), which means that certain disorders (that have always been problematic for those suffering from them) are now visible and subject to diagnosis and treatment. However, this probably applies to fewer diagnoses than the science of psychiatry would want to admit. Instead – and on the other hand – for the majority of diagnoses in the greyer area between normal human suffering and psychopathology proper, our fringe experiences in life (for want of a better word) have been psychiatrized to a considerable extent. Cultural practices and vocabularies that used to be structured around religion and morality are more and more structured around the biomedical and psychiatric complexes. This, in turn, leads to an interpretation of new forms of distress, brought about by societal transformations (first interpretation above), in a diagnostic light. Thus, we run the risk of approaching all sorts of social problems as if they were instances of individual psychopathology. The cultural-historical psychiatrization has also paved the way for the success of *Big Pharma* (and vice versa), inviting professionals and patients to see problems as locatable in the individual and her brain (third interpretation), and thus subject to psychopharmacological correction (even in the many cases where this is a deeply simplifying approach).

Finally, the fifth and last interpretation mentioned above, stemming from technical changes in the structure of diagnostic thought itself, is in its own way connected to the cultural-historical psychiatrization. My argument has been that we are building diagnostic cultures because we experience a lack of resources with which to ascribe meaning to felt suffering, so we mobilize the psychiatric-diagnostic language since it appears as something that might give meaning to our distress. The way that diagnostic psychiatry changed with the introduction of

DSM-III in 1980, however, illustrates why this is problematic and paradoxical, for moving from the etiological to the symptom-based model of diagnosis in fact served to exorcise meaning from the understanding of mental disorder. Before DSM-III, meaning was there somewhere, perhaps buried deep in the psychoanalytic unconscious, but ultimately subject to interpretation (whereby neurotic misery – in Freud's terms – could be transformed into common misery). By eliminating the meaning-giving contexts around the symptoms, modern psychiatry often reduces suffering to a mechanical reaction, in the central nervous system, for instance, instead of approaching it as a human response to an existential situation, say. Thus, meaning disappears, even if it is precisely meaning that the sufferer is looking for. The story of psychiatrization is thus in large parts a story about the loss of meaning. It is not a story of people suffering more or less, but of changed understandings of their suffering that empty their experiences of meaning. This also opens up for psychopharmacological intervention. Few would treat normal grief after the loss of a loved one with a pill, for example, but if the "reaction" is not meaningful (but simply a dysfunctional process in the brain), it might be appropriate to treat it with drugs. The cultural-historical psychiatrization (involving many sub-processes such as pathologization and pharmaceuticalization) is therefore a kind of meta-narrative that explains many of the other processes that are going on.

Four Kinds of Pathologization

All in all, it thus seems reasonable to conclude that even though society might have changed in ways that leave some people more vulnerable to experiencing distress, there is also a significant process of pathologization going on. More and more experiences, traits and conditions are looked upon in a psychiatric-diagnostic light. But it should be emphasized that pathologization is not a linear or unitary process; rather, it is made up by many, partly contradictory, processes that work in different directions at the same time. I shall here briefly name four such processes.

Stigmatization

The classic critique of pathologization, which is still warranted, states that pathologization involves stigmatizing behaviours by labelling them as ill or disordered. A stigma is a bodily mark that somehow makes the bearer visible as disgraceful. It is also associated with the stigmata, which are the wounds that resemble the crucifixion marks of Jesus. The most widespread idea of stigma in psychiatry concerns the unfair blame directed against people with various diagnosed mental problems. Few people would blame patients for having somatic health problems, but many psychiatric patients still experience society's blame and even scorn, which, of course, is appalling. Here, it is the person's behaviours that are stigmatized by society, where a diagnosis may in fact serve to reduce stigmatization, for example, by signalling a diminished capacity for autonomy and responsibility on the patient's part. The diagnosis gives access to the Parsonian "sick role" (Parsons, 1975) and, by enclosing the person's problems within a medical framework, may reduce the experienced stigma.

But stigmatization may also relate to the diagnostic category as such. It is possible to argue, for example, that diagnoses such as personality disorders are inherently stigmatizing, because they represent a blend of moral and medical discourses (Charland, 2004). Anti-social personality disorder is a psychiatric condition, but one formulated in moral terms, so, the argument goes, what happens when someone is given this diagnosis is a categorization of (morally) unwanted behaviour as pathological. Historical examples of this include the horrific stories from the Soviet Union where Stalin's psychiatrists would pathologize political dissidents in order to be able to "treat" them medically (thereby approaching them as irrational; as people that are not to be taken seriously), and also the diagnosis by the US physician Samuel Cartwright, of runaway slaves in the antebellum South with "drapetomania" (a tendency to flee the plantations, allegedly arising from overly egalitarian masters), these examples representing extreme cases of pseudo-science and scientific racism.

Fortunately, we are today a long way from these extreme kinds of pathologization as stigmatization, but it is sometimes good to bear in mind how psychiatric categories have operated in very powerful ways with serious consequences for individuals. This continues until this day, and ought to remind us just how important it is that we continuously discuss the diagnoses and their potentially stigmatizing effects.

Self-pathologization

I refer to the next form of pathologization as self-pathologization. Whereas stigmatization is a process that occurs from the outside, self-pathologization is a process in which the individual actively participates. In that sense it is a kind of reverse process to stigmatization. It can either be individuals who actively seek to have (parts of) their lives pathologized by being diagnosed, or it can be individuals, or more often collectives, who seek to have some form of suffering recognized as legitimate through the formulation of a new diagnostic category. Many of the adults that I have met as part of my fieldwork with people diagnosed with ADHD have sought out the diagnosis for themselves, and some have even paid a psychiatrist to diagnose them. (Of course, they do not pay concretely for the diagnosis, but for the assessment that often results in a diagnosis with all the benefits that may follow from this.) In a way, this testifies to the relative non-stigmatizing attitude toward ADHD, or, at least, indicates that the negative stigma that may be associated with this diagnostic category is outweighed by the positive benefits associated with being diagnosed. This is so for some diagnoses, but certainly not for all.

Different examples can illustrate how diagnoses have been formed historically in response to a felt need among the sufferers. PTSD, for example, was developed as a diagnosis that could be given to traumatized veterans from the Vietnam War (it was originally called post-Vietnam syndrome), and it was included in DSM-III in 1980. It has since become very successful as a diagnostic category, constituting part of the *lingua franca* of reactions to wars and catastrophes, as Watters puts it (Watters, 2010). Many other examples could be mentioned, for example, alcoholism, which has been transformed from a moral fault (weakness of the will) into a psychiatric problem ("Alcohol Use Disorder" in DSM-5).[1] The first step of the widespread 12-step programmes (in AA meetings, for example) is to admit that one is "powerless over alcohol – that our lives have become unmanageable", which is equivalent to suffering from some illness. Groups such as AA seem to be interested in having the problem framed as a disorder, involving a kind of collective self-pathologization. The whole range of so-called somatoform disorders (whiplash, fibromyalgia, chronic fatigue symptom and other "medically unexplained symptoms") are interesting cases in point, since patients and their organizations frequently seek self-pathologization; that is, the recognition of the problems as genuine medical issues. However, they resist *psychiatric* pathologization. These patients feel different kinds of bodily pain and are thus interested in obtaining medical diagnoses, but since there is only the subjective complaint, they are often (although it varies in different countries) referred to psychiatry, much against their will. The case is interesting, because it illustrates the problems of liminality: what happens when one's problem does not fit nicely into the established categories and disciplinary boundaries? It also illustrates the relatively low status that is still given to psychiatry in comparison with somatic diagnoses.

Risk Pathologization

Risk pathologization is the third category I shall mention, and it is in a sense pathologization *avant la lettre*. It means that one is looked upon (or that one is looking upon oneself) in pathological terms, even without manifest illness or disorder, but only because of some susceptibility to developing symptoms in the future. With the current expansion in genetic knowledge, it becomes easier and easier to determine someone's relative risk of developing a wide range of disorders where there is a genetic component involved (which there likely is in most major psychiatric problems). One should bear in mind that modern genetics are far from deterministic and that current models in genetics depict various gene-environment interaction processes that are extremely complex, and all one can get through genetic testing is some probability measure (for example of one's susceptibility to depression), but no one knows if a risk will ever materialize as a full-blown disorder.

---

1   An article from *Time* magazine estimated that around 40 per cent of all college students qualify for the diagnosis: http://healthland.time.com/2012/05/14/dsm-5-could-mean-40-of-college-students-are-alcoholics/.

So, in spite of advances in the genetic sciences, we need as human and social scientists to ask what the consequences are of living with this kind of probability knowledge. Rose talks about "the geneticization of identity" and the subsequent "genetic responsibility": "Governing oneself in the light of one's risky genes is intimately tied to identity projects, the crafting of healthy bodies, and the management of our relations with others, in relation to a wide range of authorities" (Rose, 2007, p. 126). Self-government might be enforced to an even greater degree in the future, when individuals are given the responsibility to live their lives in light of probability knowledge about their mental health. Might there even be self-fulfilling prophecies involved, such that knowing something about one's risk of developing a condition might contribute to its development? Should we protect people and give those who want it the right to *not know* about their risks? Do people have a right to "remain healthy" in the cases where they do not have serious manifest symptoms? These are questions that become increasingly pressing, and which deserve to be discussed more thoroughly in the future by psychiatrists, geneticists, philosophers and laypersons who are affected by the regimes of risk in our late modern culture.

De-pathologization

No overview of pathologization processes is complete without reference to the reverse process of de-pathologization. Again, this can refer to individuals struggling to have some diagnosis removed from them personally, but it can also refer to groups of people who fight to have some diagnosis eliminated entirely from the practices of psychiatry. Famously, homosexuality was a mental disorder according to the reigning diagnostic manuals until late in the 20th century, and it was also criminalized in many parts of the world (which is still sadly the case in some countries). It was in 1973 that Robert Spitzer (the architect of DSM-III) decided that it should not be considered a mental disorder, and this was confirmed with the publication of DSM-III in 1980 (Busfield, 2011, p. 125). However, a diagnostic category called "ego-dystonic disorder" was included, which whould apply to those who felt distress because of their homosexual orientation. Although it must be considered a breakthrough in de-pathologizing homosexuality, the new diagnosis illustrates one central problem of many psychiatric diagnoses: that forms of suffering with social origins risk being seen as individual deficiencies. For what if someone feels distressed because of his or her homosexual orientation, and what if the experienced distress is caused by a homophobic social world? The result would still be that the individual was to be diagnosed, although the problem was clearly locatable in a hostile environment. The diagnostic category of ego-dystonic disorder was removed from the DSM system in 1987, but it is still included in the WHO's ICD system and it lived on in the DSM under the heading of "sexual disorder not otherwise specified", which is characterized by "persistent and marked distress about one's sexual orientation", thereby being quite similar to the earlier formulations. Discussions and de-pathologization attempts continue to this day concerning sexuality and identity. Parts of the LGBT (lesbian, gay, bisexual, transgender) community have, for example, fought for a de-pathologization of what is otherwise diagnosable as Gender Identity Disorder or (in DSM-5) Gender Dysphoria. According to the critics of these diagnoses, it is not a disorder to identify with another gender from the one assigned at birth.

In relation to a widespread diagnosis such as ADHD, it is interesting to observe the arguments for and against. In Denmark, as in most other Western countries, there is on the one side a patient organization, the Danish ADHD Association (in the US, CHADD is an even more powerful patient organization), which works to spread knowledge and information about ADHD as a real disorder that one should take seriously. On the other side, however, there are various groups that claim that ADHD is a false disorder, nothing more than a pathologizing category, fabricated by the medical industry in order to make money. A large group in Denmark is called "ADHD is invented by Big Pharma: Stop the drugging of our children!", which has almost as many members on Facebook as the official ADHD association. The critical group organizes various happening and events and some of its members also advocate what have conventionally been seen as conspiracy theories (about the Bilderberg Group, chemtrails, a New World Order etc.). The psychiatric diagnoses, in this case ADHD, operate for groups such as this one as one symbol (among others, for some members) of an imagined enemy, around and against which one may organize. This is also a possible function of psychiatric categories in our diagnostic cultures.

Problems with Pathologization

I have tried to paint a picture of pathologization (and de-pathologization) processes as rather complex. There are many parties and stakes involved and little universal agreement as to whether psychiatric diagnoses are legitimate or illegitimately pathologizing. Only a small minority of people today argue that "Cancer is a gift" (the title of a book advocating alternative treatment) and that the medical model of this illness is misguided, but far more people are critical of the medical model of psychiatric problems and argue that (some or all of) the diagnoses pathologize. But could one not simply say "So what?", even if they do pathologize? Why is this necessarily a bad thing? I have argued in various ways in this book that diagnoses are used by individuals and groups to build and constitute identities, and why not simply accept this, *even* in those cases where it seems that there are pathologizing effects of diagnoses? As a kind of summary of some of the arguments that have been presented in previous chapters, I shall end this chapter by providing four reasons why we should in fact beware of pathologization and continue to criticize it.

(1) It easily leads to an unfair skewing of health services: this problem stems from the fact that health care and social services are part of a zero-sum game of limited resources. By stretching the concepts of diagnoses and handicaps to

encompass more and more people, fewer resources are available for those with the most severe problems (Williams, 2009). As we are witnessing a rise in diagnosed cases of anxiety, depression and ADHD in the West, we are also (at least in some countries) witnessing major problems in those sectors of psychiatry where the toughest problems are treated. As Allan Frances has argued, we spend way too much on "the worried well" and too little on the people who are suffering the most (Frances, 2013, p. xv). In my home country Denmark, there has been in the last five to ten years numerous cases of psychiatric malpractice: patients have been held for weeks and months in closed wards, and some have even died from having received too high doses of drugs. This probably does not boil down to one single cause, but it seems likely that a lack of resources in these sectors of psychiatry has something to do with it (there being insufficient beds for patients, for example, and the sector notoriously lacks doctors who specialize in psychiatry). We need to discuss whether the resources are distributed unfairly, and this involves the discussion of pathologization, for if people's ordinary life problems are pathologized, it means that there are fewer resources for those in the worst conditions. This makes the discussion of where and how to draw the line between common human suffering and pathological suffering pertinent.

(2) Pathologization processes also easily lead to what Furedi has characterized as a cultivation of vulnerability (Furedi, 2004). Naturally, this is something that mental health services would want to avoid, but today's citizens have become active consumers of diagnoses, Furedi argues, and disorders have become constitutive of people's identities. This can be called "medicalization from below" (Furedi, 2008), or what I referred to earlier as self-pathologization, although Furedi prefers to talk about psychologization, because he believes it is a process that operates through psychological categories. It nonetheless leads to people being seen as helpless and powerless, whenever they interpret themselves (and are interpreted by others) as suffering from different disorders and handicaps. If this analysis is valid, then pathologization processes come with an in-built risk of self-fulfilling prophecies, whereby people might in fact come to suffer in response to being categorized with deficit terms.

(3) Thirdly, when normal human behaviours and reactions are pathologized, people's problems are easily individualized. Instead of seeing suffering as a natural response to one's circumstances, it is seen as individual deficit or pathology. This invites the sufferers themselves, but also wider society, to approach the issue in medical terms rather than social or political terms. In order to illustrate this point, Kutchins and Kirk tell the story of a girl, who grows up in a very chaotic family which results in disruptive behaviour in school (Kutchins & Kirk, 1997). Ultimately, the girl is assessed, diagnosed with oppositional defiant disorder (ODD) and receives treatment. We can assume that the girl's unruly behaviour developed in the context of the family where she has taught herself never to trust adults (because they are *de facto* not to be trusted) and not to do what the adults tell her (because they have often told her to do things that are clearly harmful to her). In this case, the "oppositional" symptoms are actually her way of surviving

in a chaotic and problematic environment, and when these survival skills are seen as dysfunctional in the school context, it is doubly sad because the system tries to remove those few mechanisms for coping that the girl has developed and wants to retain. The problem emerges in this way, because the diagnostic system is unable to locate problems anywhere but inside the girl. Problems are individualized because of the logic of the diagnostic system, and then treatments and interventions are also often individualized. This is a major problem in our diagnostic cultures which are increasingly incapable of understanding human misery in non-diagnostic terms and intervening in non-individualist ways. It has been estimated, for example, that only ten per cent of current youthful users of hyperactivity drugs would require medication if they had "optimal family and school situations" (Horwitz, 2010, p. 94), but the preferred choice is to diagnose the individual, place the problem "inside" the person, and consequently treat this "inside" that is, in the brain.

(4) Finally, and on a more existential note, it may represent a loss of human self-understanding if we continue to pathologize more and more aspects of our lives. In the chapter on languages of suffering, I argued that our religious, existential, moral and political languages continue to be relevant to us for a number of purposes, but that these languages are often exorcised from our discussions with authorities as well as with ourselves about how our sufferings should be understood and acted upon. Even if we bracket the pragmatic issues relating to who gets access to treatment and why (which are immensely important), it is significant in its own right that we as human beings are capable of addressing our suffering adequately, which is an inescapable part of being alive as an embodied, mortal being. We ought to be able to address guilt, shame, death anxiety, broken hearts and also poverty and marginalization and so on as problems that can be experienced as painful without their being for that reason automatically transformed into mental disorders. The key – and still largely unresolved – question thus becomes: what are mental disorders, then? This is addressed in the following chapter.

Conclusions

In this chapter I have tried to interpret the diagnostic expansion that lies behind the development of diagnostic cultures. Why are more and more people categorized with psychiatric diagnoses? I presented a number of different interpretations and argued that a cultural-historical psychiatrization has taken place, where experiences, discourses and social practices have been infused with psychiatric knowledge and terminology. This is the main process that has given rise to other subordinated processes such as pharmaceuticalization and changed diagnostic practices. I then unpacked the idea of pathologization, which is a significant component in the historical processes of psychiatrization, and I argued that pathologization may move in different directions at the same time: for and against diagnoses (in the case of de-pathologization), individually and collectively, and in the direction of one specific diagnosis or several. The chapter ended by posing the "so what?" question, of why it even matters whether we think of some problem in pathological terms, which I addressed by providing four different reasons for which we need to be critical of illegitimate pathologization.

Chapter 7
Towards a Comprehensive Understanding of Mental Disorder

In this chapter I ask how we should define and approach not just psychiatric categories (diagnoses), but also the referents of diagnoses (what they are meant to refer to), which is to say mental disorders as such, from a cultural psychological perspective. First, I provide an outline of definitions of mental disorder from leading scholars (neuroscientists, Boorse, Wakefield and phenomenological perspectives), and I argue that the concept of mental disorder is not held together by necessary and sufficient conditions, but by what Wittgenstein called family resemblance. This leads to the subsequent development of a cultural psychological account of mental disorder on a non-essentialist background, which is meant to articulate a third perspective on diagnoses between essentialism and social constructionism.

What is Mental Disorder?

Those who develop new diagnostic categories and new treatments rarely discuss the difficult question: what *is* a mental disorder? That we are in fact shockingly far from being able to give a clear answer to this question is reflected in a thorough book by a leading authority on psychopathology, Derek Bolton. Bolton concludes the following:

> There is, as far as I can see, no stable reality or concept of mental disorder; it breaks up into many, quite different kinds, some reminiscent of an old idea of madness or mental illness, others nothing like this at all. (Bolton, 2008, p. viii)

Bolton thus emphasises the heterogeneity of what is conventionally called mental disorder, and, in the present context, this may serve as an indication that although some diagnostic categories may refer to genuine illnesses that are best understood as brain disorders for example (schizophrenia and bipolar disorder come to mind), others may be very different. Perhaps we should not expect that one approach to mental disorder can capture all of them. Recently, Haslam has argued:

> ... that there is little reason to believe that any one of [the] accounts of the structure of psychiatric kinds is most adequate across the board. Instead, different accounts may suit different disorders. Some psychiatric conditions may

be well described by the disease model, others by dimensional models, others by
prototype models, and so on. (Haslam, 2014, p. 13)

For a range of so-called mental disorders, we might even have reason to think that
they are not disorders at all, but rather ordinary human behaviours and reactions
that would be expected given people's circumstances. This might be the case with
conditions such as common depression, which are (mis-)interpreted as "everyday
sorrows" (Williams, 2009), social phobia (Lane, 2007) and perhaps ADHD, as I
have returned to a number of times in this book.

But let us look more closely at the notion of mental disorder. Bolton lists four
quite different overarching theories of what mental disorders are:

(1) The neuroscientific theory, according to which mental disorders express
structural or functional problems in neural processes. This theory (in different
versions) is very widespread today, especially in light of the recent renaissance
of biological psychiatry and the emergence of a human self-interpretation that has
been called "the neurochemical self" (Rose, 2007). This has led to "molecular"
interpretations of mental disorders replacing "molar" interpretations, which took
the human being as a whole into account (p. 199). I cannot do justice to the complex
discussions around neuroscience and the associated danger of reductionism, but
the main problem with the neuroscientific theory is no doubt the often weak links
between the neural and the psychological domains. Two people, both of whom
suffer from the same mental disorder, may have no brain dysfunction in common,
as there is often no one-to-one isomorphism between brain, mind and behaviour.
Furthermore, it is still the case (in spite of recent technological advances in
neuroimagery) that mental disorders are defined and identified *phenomenologically*
and *behaviourally*, and there are good principled reasons to believe that this must
remain so (Brinkmann, 2011a). Regardless of how the brain works, if a person
functions "normally", there is no reason to consider the person mentally disordered,
and there is in this sense an internal relation between mind and behaviour. This is
also what led me to be suspicious of the idea that diagnoses pick out natural kinds
in psychiatry (see Chapter 2), a suspicion that is corroborated by the current lack
of valid biomarkers with which to diagnose mental disorders. For these reasons,
the neuroscientific theory is bound to remain *auxiliary*; that is to say, it may study
the neural *correlates* of mental disorders, but this is different from studying mental
disorders *per se*, and it is therefore very unlikely that the neuroscientific theory
will ever be able to tell the whole story about mental disorders. (See also the
arguments against neuroscientific reductionism in Brinkmann, 2011b.)

(2) The medical theory, which claims that illness in general is simply a name
for subnormal functioning. This theory has been advocated with particular force by
Christopher Boorse (1976), and its aim is to provide a value-neutral understanding
of illness and health by defining disease as an internal state of the organism that
interferes with the performance of a natural function of the species (p. 62). Thus, a
mental disorder is defined as statistically subnormal functioning concerning one or
more psychological functions. The main problem with this theory is that it remains

unclear, especially when we consider *mental* disorders, what a "natural function" is. For humans, it is surely "natural" to be cultural, and there is much variety – and many divergent norms – around the world concerning normalcy and disorder (Shweder, 2008). Furthermore, for quite a few conditions (for example, mouth diseases such as caries), it seems that it is statistically normal to be ill, but without this disqualifying the conditions as illnesses. This theory therefore seems to be too simple and suffers from too many problems. Bolton mentions three: first, it is assumed that deviation from a statistical norm implies problematic functioning, which may – but need not – be the case; second, it is unclear where to draw the line between normality and disorder with reference to deviance from a mean (is it one, two or three standard deviations below the mean, for example?); and third, statistical normality is always relative to a population, but the theory does not specify which human population is the benchmark relative to which people can be said to suffer from a mental disorder (Bolton, 2008, p. 113).

(3) A third contender is Wakefield's (1992) theory of mental disorder as *harmful dysfunction*. This theory has been treated above and builds on the medical theory, but adds a *value component*. Thus, as we have seen, something is a mental disorder, according to Wakefield, if (a) the state arises because of the failure (or dysfunction) of some naturally evolved psychological mechanism that (b) affects the person in a destructive (or harmful) way; hence: disorders are harmful dysfunctions. As Wakefield makes clear, the second condition (b) implies a value judgement, since something can be judged as harmful only relative to the norms of a person's culture. An interesting consequence of this theory is that many disorders, currently listed in the DSM and ICD diagnostic systems, are in fact *not* genuine disorders. Although it is experienced as harmful, common depression, for example, is usually not the result of a malfunctioning psychological mechanism, but more often the result of social conditions that exceed the capacities of an individual, causing stress, exhaustion and eventually depression (Horwitz & Wakefield, 2005). According to Wakefield, it is therefore unwarranted to classify common depression as a mental disorder. However, the main problem with this theory is similar to the previous one: it seems quite impossible to factor out cultural from natural functions and conditions in human lives and isolate "naturally evolved psychological mechanisms", since most – if not *all* – higher mental functions depend on socialization and culture (Vygotsky, 1978). As Bolton says, it is doubtful "that there is a clear (enough) division between psychological functioning that is natural (evolved and innate), as opposed to social (cultivated)" (Bolton, 2008, p. 124).

Furthermore, Wakefield's theory seems to have some counterintuitive consequences, for *if* something is a naturally evolved function, and *if* its malfunctioning is a cause of harm for the individual, *then* it is a mental disorder, but let us return to Mubarak Bala, who we met in Chapter 1, and who allegedly suffered from a mental disorder otherwise known as *atheism*: there is some evidence from evolutionary psychology to indicate that the belief in God is the result of natural selection (Maser & Gallup, 1990) (and religious beliefs are in fact found almost universally around the globe), so if someone like Bala experiences distress because of a defective "religious module" in his evolutionarily adapted mind, his persecutors might be right to treat him! I am sure that Wakefield would not endorse this conclusion, but it does seem to follow from his account of mental disorders as harmful dysfunctions, as it is based on (quite speculative) evolutionary psychology, and thus becomes vulnerable to all sorts of discussions about which mental modules have evolved (if it is even scientifically legitimate to talk about mental modules; see the critique from biology in Sterelny, 2012).

(4) The final broad theory mentioned by Bolton is perhaps the least specific, but also in my opinion the one with the greatest appeal. This is what we might call a phenomenological theory going back to Jaspers' classical work (Jaspers, 1997), which states that mental disorders represent breakdowns in the meaningful connections and relations in our mental lives, but without the theory specifying the causes of such breakdowns. (Its focus on the experience rather than the underlying cause of the disorder is what makes it phenomenological.) If there is no traceable connection between what *happens* and how a person *reacts* (between a non-dangerous situation and anxiety, for instance), and if the person's reaction is painful and lingering, then it seems relevant to talk about a mental disorder (whether the lack of connection stems from a dysfunctional "psychological mechanism", neurological processes or whatever). This theory, which I believe holds the greatest promise (perhaps because of its lack of specificity), takes us straight to the cultural psychological issues of meaning and normativity that are invoked in this book, for when we talk about "meaningful connections", we are in the realm of norms and values. A fear of pigeons can be pathological, because there is no *reason* to fear them. A fear of poisonous snakes, on the other hand, may be rational, because they are in fact dangerous. A fear of death is surely not pathological, but may stem from the human capacity for recognizing finitude, which can be the basis for authentic, resolute living (Heidegger, 1927). So there is nothing about fear or anxiety in itself that determines its status as pathological, rational, existential or something else; rather, it depends on contextual and relational conditions of meaning. How one sees an instance of fear (and other human actions and reactions) depends on the explanatory resources that one has available.

After going through these four contenders, Bolton argues that none is satisfactory. The three kinds of naturalism represented by the neuroscientists, Boorse and Wakefield fail for different reasons, and the broader phenomenological theory might be fine as such, but it does not address the cause of the disorders, and, according to Bolton, it has the consequence that there is no meaning in mental illness (precisely because it is defined as a breakdown of meaning). Bolton rejects all essentialist accounts and argues that "there is nothing intrinsic in particular biopsychological processes that makes them pathological, it is only their consequences, only if they persistently result in more harm than good" (Bolton, 2008, p. 205). So, he wants to say that it is not the nature of the problems that people have that defines them as either psychiatric, social, moral, existential or something else (cf. the chapter on languages of suffering); rather, it is our *response* to the problems. This, I find, is also not satisfactory, since it appears to be circular, because we (and here I include not only researchers, but also the systems of treatment at large) want to know *how* to approach people's problems. As such, we need some sort of guidance concerning how to do that *before* we make a response. We would also like to know when someone is fit for the rule of law, and when he or she is mentally ill, which might necessitate the insanity defence (Robinson, 1996). Bolton's alternative seems to be that it is in the eyes of the beholder – that is, in our response to the problem – that the matter is decided, and this quickly leads to a social constructionist deconstruction of the idea of mental disorder as such, because then we could simply choose *not* to respond to the problem as one of mental illness – and that would surely eliminate mental disorders – or would it?

I what follows I have no intention of settling this thorny issue once and for all, but I do wish to investigate whether cultural psychology can help us find a way between naturalist essentialisms (which are misguided for the reasons listed by Bolton) and social constructionist disbandings of ideas of mental disorders as such. However, I believe that this might presuppose that we give up the attempt to find necessary and sufficient conditions for something to count as a mental disorder (and here I am in agreement with Bolton), and instead insist that the concept is held together by family resemblance, to borrow a term from Wittgenstein (1953). Wittgenstein famously analysed concepts such as "game" and demonstrated that there is not one thing that all games have in common, which is what makes them games, just as there need not be one thing that all members of a family share (such as eye colour) in order for them to be members of the same family. Similarly, it is quite likely that the concept of mental disorder is characterized by fuzzy boundaries and different characteristics that criss-cross, without there being one defining feature that they all share (Lilienfield & Marino, 1995).

Toward a Cultural Psychological Alternative

Cultural psychology, in the version articulated in this book, is today a significant approach in general psychology and many related fields and disciplines, but it is curious to notice how little today's cultural psychology has to say about mental disorder, which is otherwise a key theme in psychology as a whole. In many people's eyes, it is probably even the case that psychology's *raison d'être* lies in its ability to help us understand and treat mental disorder. Most theorizing on mental disorder in psychology has historically been dominated by psychodynamic, cognitivist and behaviourist schools, and more recently by the neurosciences. It is well known that Vygotsky (considered by many to be a founding father of cultural psychology) took a significant interest in abnormal psychology in children, or "defectology" as it was then called (Vygotsky, 1929), but browsing through today's authoritative sources on cultural psychology, such as *The Cambridge Handbook of Sociocultural Psychology* (Valsiner & Rosa, 2007), leaves one with the impression that an interest in mental disorder and distress, particularly in adults, is more or less non-existent. This is probably an unfair verdict, and there are certainly interesting studies of mental disorder here and there by cultural psychologists, but they do not in any way define the field, and no well-developed theoretical account of mental disorder exists in cultural psychology today.

In the remainder of this chapter, I begin to articulate a theoretical account of mental disorder from a cultural psychological perspective. It is argued that cultural psychology has the potential to develop a comprehensive understanding of mental disorder that combines awareness of the brain and body with sociocultural norms and practices without reducing mental disorder to either of these. In that sense, it may steer a course between essentialist models of psychopathology on the one hand, and radical social constructionist ones on the other. Attention deficit hyperactivity disorder (ADHD) in adults is once more referred to as an illustrative example, but the theory presented here has more general ambitions. Following the convention in much of the clinical literature, I begin by introducing a case of a person who has been diagnosed with a mental disorder (ADHD), before venturing into a more theoretical landscape.

Tom's Story

In order to have a concrete case to use as a springboard for the ensuing discussions, I shall introduce Tom. I first met Tom in the summer of 2013, when I began my fieldwork as a participant observer in a support group for adults diagnosed with ADHD. I still participate in the group as of 2015, which meets for about three hours once every month. Tom is there almost every time, and I have also interviewed him in his home. I do this fieldwork in order to understand how adults diagnosed with ADHD use the diagnosis in their own lives. They are not simply given the diagnosis as passive recipients, but actively are use it for a number of purposes. The ADHD category operates as a powerful semiotic mediator in their lives that enables them to interpret their past in a new light and develop specific hopes and possible developmental pathways for the future, while excluding others (see Chapter 4). I am interested in the phenomenological aspects of being diagnosed – how do people experience this process? – and also in how the diagnosis is used discursively by those who come to "live under the description" of ADHD, to borrow Emily Martin's terminology (Martin, 2007). Most of the people in the group (there are usually around 15 people present at a meeting) have sought out the diagnosis themselves, either because their children have been diagnosed (and they see themselves mirrored in the children's problems), or because they have been through some sort of crisis in their lives (such as a stress related breakdown) that prompted a more thorough examination by the doctor and later the psychiatrist, which eventually led to the ADHD diagnosis. This is quite unlike the situation for children diagnosed with ADHD, who are very rarely (if ever) the ones who initiate a diagnostic process.

Tom, a man living alone in his mid-forties, also wanted the diagnosis himself. When he told his life story in an interview with me, he talked about a history of unruly behaviours, concentration problems, and also petty crimes in his late teenage years. He was adopted as a small child after having spent the first month of his life at an orphanage, and he talked repeatedly about his quite strong temper. He received no ADHD diagnosis during his years at school; he was simply seen as one of the "naughty boys". After school, he was able to hold down a number of jobs, still has good friends, and he also used to have a girlfriend, with whom he lived. He describes himself as "an ADHD person who is functioning well". He seems quite determined in his choices and opinions. For example, when he discovered that there was a long waiting list before he could see the psychiatrist and obtain a diagnosis (paid for by the state), he decided to pay for the psychiatric assessment out of his own pocket, and he was finally given the ADHD diagnosis about six months before I met him for the first time. He is still in a process of reading and learning about the diagnosis and trying to adjust his medicine to an optimal level. He grows his own marijuana, which he consumes occasionally (but does not sell to others), and psychiatrists would probably see this as "self-medication". He is currently unemployed, but, interestingly, his last job was as a support person for young people with various problems, many of whom also have an ADHD diagnosis, so he now knows the diagnosis both as a professional and as a patient.

Tom's story is in some ways typical (concerning his history and problems as a child, for example), but in other ways it is (like all life stories) unique. When interviewing Tom in his apartment, eating cake and drinking coffee, I remember very clearly that I had the thought that this person is not mentally disordered. So why was he given the diagnosis? What does it tell us about our current diagnostic cultures, in which more and more conditions are seen through the diagnostic lens, that Tom received a psychiatric diagnosis? Two things about Tom's situation are particularly noteworthy in this context, and I shall use these as background information in the following discussion about the concept of mental disorder and how to approach this in cultural psychological terms.

First, Tom is a very organized person. His apartment is perfectly clean and tidy, and he has neat to-do lists placed on the refrigerator. He had prepared carefully for the interview with me, for example, by reading from a book on adult ADHD authored by a well-known Danish psychiatrist and a psychologist, and he had written down a summary of its central messages that he wanted to show me in order to convey what ADHD feels like for him. The capability of organizing his life and daily projects goes against the diagnostic criteria for ADHD, where having "trouble organizing tasks and activities" and "is often forgetful in daily activities" are central. Tom is aware of this himself, but explained it by saying that "it is in order to avoid the chaos" that he has a high level of organization. In other words, he compensates so well – by using calendars and to-do-lists, and perhaps also his marijuana – that many of the symptoms of disorganization in fact disappear. The crucial question then becomes: if the symptoms disappear, is the diagnosis still warranted? As I have described in this book, diagnostic psychiatry has since 1980 (with the introduction of DSM-III) been based on an assessment of symptoms (rather than on an understanding of the etiology and underlying psychodynamics of the person), so, strictly speaking, it means that a disorder is only there if and when the symptoms are present (Horwitz, 2002). Paradoxically, this seems to imply that people's compensatory actions will remove the pathology.

Second, Tom described how his problems really emerged after an injury he suffered while he was in the armed forces. He was on a three-year contract and wanted to make a career in the military, but his leg was more or less crushed in a traffic accident, and he had to leave the military. Tom described the forces as a very good place to work, and it seems evident that the symptoms of ADHD were not present in his life during this period. So, the next question (which is related to the former) becomes: did Tom in fact have ADHD when he was in the military? Is it possible to have ADHD in an extremely organized context with clear hierarchies and task allocations? Do the social practices of the military provide an ecological niche, to use Hacking's (1998) term, in which the cognitive problems otherwise associated with ADHD are eliminated?

The point of raising these questions is to demonstrate that how one answers them will depend on the theory of mental disorder to which one (implicitly or explicitly) subscribes. Two of the essentialist theories included above (the neuroscientific and Boorse's statistical theory) would likely say that Tom has always had ADHD, because of his brain and suboptimal level of functioning. Wakefield's theory would say that even if Tom has a psychological dysfunction, this only becomes ADHD the moment that it is "harmful". So, although this theory is also essentialist (because of its focus on the alleged dysfunctional mental module within the person), it also has a contextual or cultural component. The phenomenological theory is harder to apply to Tom's case, because it seems misguided to say that there is a breakdown in the otherwise meaningful connections in his life.

Moving to a more metatheoretical level, we can group the various positions together and say that there are essentialist and social constructionist positions: essentialists on the one side would say that if one has ADHD, then one has ADHD all the time and everywhere, because the disorder is constituted by certain core neurocognitive deficits, while on the other side, most social constructionists (which were not included among Bolton's theories, because they more or less repudiate the very concept of mental disorder) would say that ADHD is a socially constructed category that medicalizes and pathologizes problematic behaviours, and such social constructionists would thereby seek to deconstruct all pathological "essences" associated with the diagnosis. I shall explicate these divergent standpoints further in what follows, before articulating a cultural psychological theory that is neither essentialist nor social constructionist (in a radical sense), but rather situational, relational, and mediational, and thus, I shall argue, more theoretically sound.

Essentialist and Constructionist Approaches to Mental Disorder

According to a number of leading analysts that have also been referred to in this book, contemporary understandings of mental disorder in the West are heavily influenced by 'biomedicalization' (Clarke & Shim, 2010). Despite the fact that no simple biomarkers have been found for any mental disorder in psychiatry (Singh & Rose, 2009), and even though diagnoses can only be formulated by evaluating and counting symptoms (and not through brain scans or blood tests), there is a huge interest among researchers in the neuroscience of mental disorder that trickles down to the public and its "folk psychiatry". My argument is not that the brain is unimportant in relation to mental disorders (quite the contrary), but I simply wish to point out that it is not possible to diagnose any mental disorder by looking at a person's brain. The enormous interest in the neurosciences of mental disorder these years (depicted and analyzed in Rose & Abi-Rached, 2013) has gone hand in hand with the success of *Big Pharma*, if not concerning the treatment of mental disorder (where the results are mixed to put it mildly, as discussed in the previous chapter), but rather in the marketing and spread of pharmaceuticals for treating a number of conditions such as anxiety, depression and ADHD. Today, the pharmaceutical industry is among the largest in the world with marketing budgets that are twice as large as the money they spend on research and development of new drugs (Frances, 2013).

Concerning ADHD specifically, the now standard account in psychiatry is one that approaches this condition as a neurocognitive deficit, resulting in inattention, impulsivity, and hyperactivity to varying degrees, which are seen as chronic symptoms that can be treated with stimulant medicine, but which can never be cured (Buitelaar, Kan & Asherson, 2011). The neuroscientific approach easily (however not necessarily) invites researchers to think in essentialist terms and look for the core dysfunctional brain mechanism that is thought to be involved in ADHD. Scores of brain imaging studies are now published every year, which are interpreted in the light of quite different theoretical paradigms. Some theories follow Russell Barkley who states that ADHD is at its core a disorder of behavioural inhibition (Barkley, 1997), while others are in agreement with Thomas Brown, who argues that the deficit lies in the inner management system of attention (Brown, 2005). Maiese (2012) provides a very helpful comparative discussion of these essentialist models and their respective shortcomings. In either case, the ambition is to be able to pinpoint exactly what the alleged deficit is in essentialist terms. Perhaps ADHD is even a natural kind, some will say; that is, a specific illness "entity" that can be defined in terms of necessary and jointly sufficient properties (see Chapter 2), which ideally leads to a "strict in or out classification of all individuals" (Kincaid & Sullivan, 2014, p. 3). This, at least, seems to be the essentialists' dream, which, if realized, would likely lead to more valid diagnoses linked directly to the brain rather than behavioural symptoms.

Among a number of problems related to essentialism, I shall merely mention two. First, as I have already pointed out, no "essences" (in the sense of simple biomarkers) have in fact been found in psychiatry as a whole, let alone in relation to ADHD. Essentialism rests on what the historian of medicine Charles Rosenberg has called disease specificity (see Chapter 2), which refers to the idea that diseases are specific entities that have a kind of independent existence beyond their unique manifestations in sick individuals (Rosenberg, 2007, p. 13). To repeat Rosenberg's point: before the 19th century, there were sick people, and after there emerged actual diseases. Although the idea of disease specificity might apply to somatic medicine, where examples such as cancer or diabetes can serve as obvious illustrations, it seems quite problematic in psychiatry (Frances, 2013, p. 19).

Second, and possibly even more detrimental to essentialism, is the sociological insight that disorders "are only intelligible due to the normative and social context in which they are found" as Bowden has recently argued (Bowden, 2014, p. 422). Among philosophers of psychiatry today, there is widespread agreement that one cannot define anything as a disorder in the absence of social norms of normality and suffering (Horwitz & Wakefield, 2007). Even if we grant that what is today referred to as ADHD is a ubiquitous trait in human populations across time and place (as some evolutionary psychologists will say; see Bolton, 2008), we still need social norms in order to establish whether this trait represents a disorder or is simply "a way of being human".

Such arguments have led some to the belief that all mental disorders are nothing more or less than contingent social constructions. This, obviously, is the antithesis to essentialist accounts, which is often referred to as social constructionism. Social constructionist models of disorder dissolve essentialist definitions and claim that the whole range of problematic human behaviours represent disorders only because of social categorizations and not because of anything inherent in the people who suffer. Social constructionist models come in many versions that are more or less epistemologically and metaphysically radical, but they all seem to "encourage the view that social values and priorities are the sole historical determinants of medicine, music, and marriage", as Church writes in her account of social constructionist approaches to mental disorder (Church, 2004, p. 393). Some, like Kenneth Gergen, seemingly prefer to eliminate the "deficit discourse" of mental disorder entirely, as this is incarnated in the diagnostic vocabulary (Gergen, 1994), while others, such as the less radical Peter Conrad, argue that diagnosing people with the ADHD category is a species of medicalization that amounts to "social control" (Conrad, 2006). The point is that abnormal behaviours, such as the deviance labelled as ADHD, "is not inherent to the individual, the act, or the situation, but [is] rather a process in which certain alleged 'rule-breaking' actions come to be defined as deviance" (p. 1). In other words, for a social constructionist, there are no mental disorders "out there"; they are all in the eyes of the pathologizing beholder.

If the essentialists tend to forget that social norms are needed to establish anything as a mental disorder, it can be argued that the social constructionists conversely tend to forget that suffering individuals very often look for "pathologizations" to explain their problems. This was the case in Tom's story recounted above. Tom wanted the diagnosis himself, because he lacked an explanation of his problems. With their eagerness to move beyond the individual to the social context, social constructionists fail to acknowledge not only that individuals may bring quite different problems *into* a context, but also that individuals may in fact be very positive toward the deficit discourses that social constructionists wish to eliminate for the sake of the diagnosed.

It seems simplistic to say that ADHD, for example, is nothing but a matter of social control, just as it seems like a naïve dream to look for a never-changing "ADHD essence" in the brains of the diagnosed. To return to Tom, it is noteworthy that he has not had his brain scanned, and it is quite unlikely (although we do not know this for sure) that anything about his brain would appear abnormal. In any case, he functions relatively well in his everyday life. It also seems far-fetched to understand his problems in terms of social control. He does have a history of problems, which, however, have waxed and waned as he has moved through different life contexts. At the same time, we no doubt need to take both social norms and practices into account when seeking to understand him and other people diagnosed with ADHD, together with the fact that these persons have brains and bodies that appear in certain ways (for example the restless movements of hands and feet that are characteristic of many people with the diagnosis) and are affected by the drugs in ways that many people (including Tom) appreciate. (Almost all the people with the ADHD diagnosis that I have met in my fieldwork use drugs such as methylphenidate and generally praise their effects, although there are exceptions.) In my view, there is a need for an integrative understanding of mental disorders such as ADHD that is able to incorporate all these dimensions, and which steers a course between essentialism and constructionism. We need a theory that can take into account the fact that our representations and categorizations of people influence how they experience and act in relation to their problems, but which at the same time acknowledges that their problems are not simply created by the fact that we categorize them. I believe that this is where cultural psychology is well-positioned to assist with its broad theoretical outlook. The rest of this chapter provides an outline of how a cultural psychology of mental disorder may look; based on a theory of illness as situated. The outline is theoretical and future work is needed to articulate its methodological implications, which, I believe, should rest on (qualitative) approaches that are able to grasp a person's mediated life in its totality, including an awareness of how discourses and categories meet and intermingle with bodily experiences and social contexts. (See Nielsen, 2015; Rønberg, 2015, for qualitative studies of ADHD and depression that move in this direction.)

A Situational Approach to Mental Disorders

The Danish medical sociologist Dorte Gannik (who sadly died much too early in 2012) devoted much of her career to developing a situational theory of illness, which I have found to be deeply congenial to cultural psychology (Gannik, 2005; 2009). Her work, which was based on studies of somatic illness, notably back problems, is little known outside Scandinavia, but her theory is noteworthy because of its simple elegance. While it is certainly relevant in relation to somatic medicine, it seems to be even more to the point concerning psychiatric problems.

For reasons similar to those articulated above, Gannik rejected essentialist theories of illness and disease (although there is a conventional distinction between illness and disease, this is rendered problematic by her theory), sseeing illness as something relational, "identical with a person's interactive relationship with her surroundings", and also as performative: "The theory abstains from approaching illness as something 'in itself' beyond those actions or reactions with which a person responds to everyday, bodily experiences (Gannik, 2005, p. 332). Referring to the well-established fact that symptoms are pervasive in our lives and that most of us experience unpleasant sensations in our bodies every day, Gannik made the point that symptoms are not diseases or disorders, arguing that we should talk about illness, disease or disorder as something people "do" (perform, enact) in relation to physical and social environments. They exist only in and through the ways in which they are performed. This has also been argued by the ethnographer and philosopher Annemarie Mol, in her study of atherosclerosis, for example (Mol, 2002). Mol says that we should not think of diseases as "constructed", since this metaphor solely emphasizes human symbolic activities of social construction, thereby leaving out the body and the material world (p. 32). Instead we should use the metaphor of performance, or talk about "enactment". Objects such as disorders are enacted in practices, but this should not lead us to the view that they are simply done by discrete actors (who could just choose to do otherwise). Instead, the idea of enactment suggests "that activities take place – but leaves the actors vague" (p. 33). Enactments presuppose a whole range of mediators that make the doing possible. If we ask: "Who does the doing?" (of ADHD, for instance), then the answer has to include not just the suffering person, for events "are made to happen by several people and lots of things. Words participate, too. Paperwork. Rooms, buildings. The insurance system" (p. 25). And much more. The complexity involved leads to a need for what Mol calls a "praxiographic appreciation of reality" (p. 53), which studies how things are brought into being in socio-material practices. (I refer the reader to her book to get an idea of how to work methodologically with this perspective.) *Contra* essentialism, this means that it becomes impossible to isolate the "essence" of a disorder in any one place (such as the brain), and, *contra* social constructionism, it means that many forces besides the purely human (such as symbolic or discursive) ones are involved.

Returning to Gannik, we can say that her model likewise does not isolate illness/ disorder in anything in the person as such (essentialism), or in anything in the social system in itself (constructionism). Rather, illness and disorder are always found in a *relation* between a person (or organism) and life situations (constituted by socio-material practices). This relational perspective means that people's problems are radically situated. They exist in their concretely situated manifestations only, and not in anything behind or beyond this. Thus, essentialism fails. But it also means that the problems are irreducibly real – as real as anything gets – and sometimes stubbornly real. Thus, social constructionism in its radical versions fails. We should maintain a moderate social constructionist outlook, because certain important factors related to mental disorder are socially constructed (some norms inherent in our social practices, for instance), but we should also acknowledge the importance of factors that cannot be said to be socially constructed. It is the *relation* between these factors that should be in focus. Gannik's theory implies that treating people's disorders relationally may involve changing the person (for example, through cognitive techniques or drugs) or changing the socio-material practices (for example, by inventing new cultural prosthetic devices or new discursive practices). The point is that someone's problems are not to be located in a single place, but dispersed over multiple mediators.

If we look at Tom's story through this lens, we can see that his problems are not just socially constructed, and it seems unhelpful to claim that the ADHD diagnosis in this case is merely a species of social control (*pace* Conrad, 2006). There is felt suffering in his life, related to disruptive behaviours and a problematic temper, but, at the same time, this phenomenon seems to become ADHD only in the context of certain socio-material practices and their norms, relative to which the problem can be enacted as ADHD. A cultural psychology of mental disorders should ask what mediators are involved in a given case that makes this form of enactment possible. (I provide a sketchy answer below.)

A situational approach to Tom's story also seems to imply that in certain contexts, such as the military, where the "symptoms" are not enacted, we should beware of concluding that he "has ADHD". Perhaps we need to conclude that Tom did *not* have ADHD in the military. From the situational perspective, one does not simply "have" ADHD (or any other disorder) – here, there and everywhere – but enacts it only when certain contextual conditions and mediators are present, and even in life contexts where the condition can be enacted (such as in schools), we see someone like Tom being able to remove or at least diminish his symptoms with the use of culturally available technologies such as to-do lists. As a cultural psychologist, one may hope that future research into ADHD and related diagnoses does not only aim to develop new drugs to target brain chemistry, but also the much more immediately significant (yet with much less prestige and money involved) everyday artefacts that may be used as cognitive "assistive technologies" (Gillespie, Best & O'Neill, 2012).

The Mediated Mind and Its Disorders

If we follow Gannik and Mol and look for a framework between essentialism and radical constructionism, the question for a cultural psychologist becomes: what kinds of mediators are involved in making the enactment of a given disorder possible? And the practice-oriented question becomes: how can these mediators be changed in order to help persons who suffer? Using the term "mediator" in this way obviously draws upon the tradition in cultural psychology of seeing the mind (and its disorders) as mediated. In Chapter 1, I introduced a cultural psychological theory of the mind as a set of skills and dispositions, constituted by different sets of mediators, and in previous general psychological publications (Brinkmann, 2011b;

2012), I have developed this theory by arguing (1) that psychological phenomena (our ways of acting, feeling, perceiving, and thinking) are normative in the sense that they do not simply happen, but are rather done (performed, enacted) by persons relative to social norms inherent in social practices (see also Harré, 2002); (2) that the mind should be thought of not as an entity, but as a name for the skills and dispositions that enable persons to enact psychological phenomena; and (3) that a range of mediators are involved in the constitution of this enactment. Some of the mediators are literally tools, while others, such as the brain, can be thought of metaphorically as tools (Harré, 2012). The four major kinds of mediators are the brain, the body, social practices, and material artefacts, as depicted below in Figure 7.1. I shall briefly discuss how these (which overlap and criss-cross) may each be involved in the constitution of the ADHD phenomenon. Needless to say, I can only provide a sketch of the argument in this context.

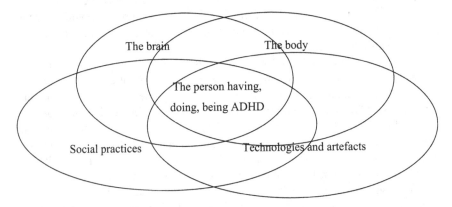

Figure 7.1   The mediators constituting the phenomenon of ADHD

Concerning the brain, it must be said that although no biomarkers for ADHD (or any other mental disorder) have been found that make diagnosis possible, it is inconceivable for most researchers (including me) that the brain is not involved in constituting the ADHD phenomenon, for the simple reason that the central nervous system is active in relation to any psychological process imaginable. The brain is a tool that persons employ when they think, feel and act – and also when they fail to do so in culturally sanctioned ways. A reductionist programme in the neurosciences will study how thinking, feeling and acting go on in the brain, but a cultural psychologist (who is open to the neurosciences) will rather insist that only *persons* (and not their brains) think, feel and act (sometimes in ways that are labelled 'ADHD'), although they definitely need their brains to do so. Large research programmes now investigate the brains of people with the ADHD diagnosis (Buitelaar, Kan & Asherson, 2011), and we will have to wait and see whether something significant emerges. (We know that the brain is plastic, which may mean that no common pattern – or essence – can be found in the brain across people diagnosed.) In any case (and I consider this a quite trivial point), the brain is without doubt a mediator that is involved in constituting the ADHD phenomenon.

This also goes for the body. Not many researchers are concerned with the embodied nature of mental disorders, but Maiese (2012) is one exception in the case of ADHD. Based on a phenomenology of the body, she argues that ADHD represents a problematic bodily orientation through which a person interacts with and gives meaning to the world. She further argues that embodied affective framing mechanisms, which serve to help people understand what is important in different situations, are defective in people who suffer from ADHD. It is difficult to assess the degree to which this perspective applies to Tom, particularly because the ways in which he has organized himself in his home render his everyday life predictable, but from meetings and conversations with many other adults diagnosed with ADHD, it is recognizable that some of them have trouble focusing on what for most other people is salient in a social situation (which sometimes leads to curious interpersonal misunderstandings). Some researchers have also noted the bodily asynchronicity and lack of "social rhythm" that characterizes some people with the ADHD diagnosis, and this is something that calls for further research into embodiment and not just neuroscience.

Thirdly, and almost trivially from a social scientific perspective, is the way that ADHD is mediated by certain social norms as they are inscribed into social practices. Researchers have found, for example, that a child's date of birth is a very powerful predictor of whether or not that child will receive the ADHD diagnosis: studies from the US show that a boy born in January has a 70 per cent higher risk of being diagnosed than a boy born in December, owing to the cut-off date for being assigned to a school grade (Frances, 2013, p. 141). What happens is that a child's relatively immature behaviours are pathologized as ADHD within the social practices of today's schools. With this, of course, I do not mean to imply that children really have ADHD because of their date of birth, but this finding certainly makes it evident that ADHD is co-constituted by norms about concentration and unobtrusiveness in modern society and specifically schools. In his account of the historical creation of ADHD, the historian Matthew Smith has even gone so far as to link the hyperactivity epidemic in the US with the "*Sputnik* panic" that emerged after the Russians succeeded in launching *Sputnik* in orbit around the Earth, leading panicked American educators to reform US schools in order to be able to beat the Soviet Union, which allegedly had much more discipline when compared to the reform pedagogy of John Dewey that had otherwise characterized the American school system (Smith, 2012). It is fascinating that global politics might in this way lead to very local consequences for individuals who are diagnosed. For Tom, as I have tried to demonstrate, it is quite clear that his symptoms appear as problematic only outside the strongly organized context of the military, where he has had to lead an independent adult life, deciding every day what is to be done, when, and how. Modern life in the West has been described as involving a "tyranny of choice" (Schwartz, 2004), celebrating the autonomous, reflective decision-maker in numerous social practices, and this may create ecological niches in which people are prone to being diagnosed with ADHD if they do not live up to the norms of constant free choice. Obviously, this also presupposes that the very category exists, which has been the case in the DSM system since 1987.

Finally, the fourth kind of mediator is the artefactual, involving all kinds of technologies. For some disorders, it is obvious that mediators of this kind are involved in the constitution of the problem: dyslexia, for example, is only possible because of the existence of written language. Concerning ADHD, it is interesting that the diagnostic criteria include such things as "fidgets with or taps hands or squirms in seat" and "loses things necessary for tasks or activities (e.g., school materials, pencils, books, tools, wallets, keys, paperwork, eyeglasses and mobile telephones)".[1] In a world without seats (in school institutions), pencils, books etc. (which are representatives of "learning technologies" as such), and without the relevant socio-material arrangements of educational practices in which bodies are socialized to a certain type of behaviour, it is difficult to imagine that ADHD could exist. Technologies may assist in the creation of disorders, but may of course also help alleviate symptoms, and I have already described how material technologies are used by Tom in attempts to regulate his life activities in various fruitful ways.

The point of listing these is to emphasize that the disorder cannot be isolated to any one of these sets of mediators, but must be seen as distributed between and across them. The argument is that there is no essence anywhere that makes up ADHD in and of itself, but different mediators (neuronal, bodily, practical, discursive and artefactual) may be relationally involved in different cases to constitute a problem as one of ADHD. Together, the mediators enable persons to enact their problems as ADHD: a working brain and body are needed, as are social practices with norms and discursive categories, and also various artefacts (and I have not gone into detail concerning the technologies of symptom checklists, pills, smartphone apps etc.). Talking about enacting ADHD – or living under the description of "ADHD" (Martin, 2007) – is not to say that people do so consciously. Behaviours that we designate as ADHD are not chosen, but they are also not completely mechanical. I agree with Martin (who talks about bipolar disorder in the following quote) that being hyperactive "does not fit easily at either end of opposites like conscious/ unconscious, habitual/novel; compelled/chosen; or innate/learned" (p. 83). We need a new language, a new scientific approach to "describe the terrain between these poles" (p. 83), since this is where most disorders are enacted. Moving into this terrain should be a task for cultural psychologists, if they want to study mental disorder, and they are particularly well equipped to do so because of their broad, holistic approach to mental life.

My argument can be summed up by returning briefly to Tom. If my argument is valid, we should see Tom's ADHD as mediated by his brain, body, social practices and various technologies. *Contra* essentialism, his problems are not restricted to any one of these, and, *contra* constructionism, ADHD represents more than a

---

1   http://www.cdc.gov/ncbddd/adhd/diagnosis.html

(pathologizing) discourse that is applied to a neutral or formless world. Hopefully, a cultural psychological broadening of our approaches to mental disorder can also lead to innovative and humane ways of helping people with their problems. Sometimes, the best help is likely to be found by looking at a few of the mediators (perhaps just a single one), but I shall claim that in principle we should be able to address all of them. Cultural psychologists are particularly well equipped to study the mediators of social practices and technologies, but they should also be sensitive to the embodied nature of mental problems. It could be objected that Tom is a special case, and that other disorders manifest themselves much more systematically in people's lives. This is probably correct, but I do not think that it invalidates the general argument that cultural psychologists should theorize mental disorders as enacted relational, situational problems, related to a mediated mind.

There is often an element of choice involved in the designation of human problems. It is not clear-cut that the most adequate approach to Tom's is one that conceives of his problem as a mental disorder. This is quite often the case and represents a challenge to the major theories of mental disorder: against the neuroscientific theory, we must say that we really do not know if there is anything "wrong" with Tom's brain, and we do not know which brain represents normality anyway; *contra* Boorse's theory we can say that yes, it is likely that Tom sub-performs statistically on some parameters related to concentration and impulse control, but if these problems are only made manifest in certain environments, it seems to be overly individualistic to isolate the problem within him; against Wakefield's theory, we must reply that it seems to be quite speculative to argue that Tom has a dysfunctional mental module (and how should this be assessed in practice anyway?); and, finally, *contra* the phenomenological approach, we find it hard to pinpoint a "breakdown in meaningful connections" in Tom's life. But, still, he does have his problems – especially since leaving the military – and my argument has been that it is better to give up the search for one single theory about mental disorder and instead recognize the different sets of mediators that are in play to make the enactment of ADHD possible for him. It is likely that an awareness of this will also enable Tom and others around him to improve his life conditions and perhaps eliminate the symptoms of ADHD, as was the case in his military years.

Conclusions

In this chapter I have looked directly at the notion of mental disorder and tried to develop a comprehensive approach based on an integrative cultural psychological theory. According to this theory, mental disorders are generally not constituted by necessary and sufficient conditions, they are not natural kinds (cf. Chapter 2), and there are no essences (for instance, in the brain) that in and of themselves make up mental disorders. As such we need a non-essentialist theory, but this does not mean that we should conclude that talk of mental disorders is "just" a discourse that generates what it talks about. A rejection of essentialism should not lead us to a radical social constructionist position. Discourses and categories are important (particularly as boundary objects holding practices together; see Bowker & Star, 2000), but they represent merely one kind of force that becomes entangled with other kinds of forces – related to brains, bodies and environments – to constitute mental disorders. This, in short, is a situational and relational perspective on the mind and its disorders that was developed with reference to Gannik (and also Mol). As boundary objects, diagnoses represent and refer to "hybrids of nature and culture, and technohuman complexes" (Lock, 2001, p. 488), and the disorders of the mind are not – just as the mind itself is not – "located in any one place at all but is rather distributed among the brain, the body and the environment", as the phenomenological psychiatrist and theoretician of psychopathology Thomas Fuchs has argued (Fuchs, 2009, p. 221). So, the cultural psychological analysis does not deny that there are neural components to mental problems, but simply (which, however, is not so simple!) insists that something can become manifest as a mental disorder only in sociocultural practices where embodied *persons* act, think and feel (sometimes in problematic ways). Diagnoses, experiences and disorders are entangled in complex ways and are just as much properties of the environment as they are of the organism.

Few studies have so far applied this perspective empirically, but an exception is the study of stress as a collective and distributed phenomenon in the workplace by Kirkegaard and Brinkmann (2015). In psychology, stress is now often conceived on the model introduced by Lazarus (Lazarus & Folkman, 1984), according to which stress develops on the basis of two cognitive steps, the first of which involves the question of whether a happening in a person's life is a threat or not, and the second being concerned with an appraisal of one's resources for coping with that happening (if it is indeed assessed as a threat). Based on fieldwork in a work organization, Tanja Kirkegaard has demonstrated that the processes of appraisal and coping are on the one hand much more socially embedded than Lazarus' original formulations made it seem. One rarely appraises and copes in isolation, but rather among and with others with whom one is in dialogical engagements. And, of course, the processes are also situated in a material landscape of offices, calendars, computers, meetings and much more that constitute resources (and barriers) in persons' attempts at coping with their tasks and threats. Thus, if this study is valid and potentially generalizable, it can inspire us to rethink not only stress (which is not as such a psychiatric diagnosis), but also other mental problems in distributed, dialogical and relational terms. Stress, ADHD, depression and all the other mental problems are *experienced, had* and *done* by persons, but this does not mean that the problems can be isolated to what goes on "within" the person. Numerous other factors are at work, including the effects of diagnostic categories as such.

Chapter 8
General Conclusions

As I put it in the introduction to this book, my aims in this book have been fourfold:

(1) To chart the emerging diagnostic cultures in contemporary society and ask: how do psychiatric diagnoses affect modern society and the people living today?

(2) To analyze the impact of diagnostic cultures on our understanding of and coping with various human problems: how are diagnoses put to use by individuals who are diagnosed (or increasingly understand themselves in light of diagnostic categories)?

(3) To articulate a cultural psychological perspective (integrating social psychology, sociology and cultural studies) that is applicable to "clinical" phenomena (such as ADHD): how do personal problems interact with broader societal trends, and how can this be studied?

(4) To critically question the distinction between nature and culture, or biology and the social sciences, which is increasingly incapable of helping us explain the sufferings that people feel in their lives today: if most mental disorders that are diagnosed represent entanglements of biological, psychological and social issues, then how should mental disorder be defined and addressed (theoretically and in practice)?

I shall now return to these aims and questions and summarize how I have approached them throughout the book. I shall do so under a set of headings that I believe capture some of the most important dilemmas and concerns in our diagnostic cultures, which have appeared across the different chapters in this book.

Problems and Potentials in Diagnostic Cultures

How do psychiatric diagnoses affect modern society and the people living today? That was my first question, and I have in this book pointed to a large number of functions of the diagnoses. For a complex modern society and its welfare institutions, diagnoses represent a significant allocation tool that is used to distribute resources for treatments, interventions, and welfare benefits and services. For health professionals and researchers, diagnoses are often the starting point that must be made clear before other things are known about a patient, whilst for the diagnosed themselves – who have been in focus in the book – psychiatric diagnoses are used to frame their problems as forces or entities (cf. "entification") within persons, which may be controllable or not. They are used in a moral economy of blaming and excusing, and first and foremost they are used to provide explanations for people's sufferings and eccentricities, whether this is theoretically warranted or not. Although I have often been critical of the functions of diagnoses in this book, I have also tried to look at their benefits, which is a general trend today, as researchers are interested in both positive and negative aspects of psychiatric diagnoses (McGann, 2011, p. 332).

Chapter 3 showed how human suffering can be conceptualized and acted upon with the use of different languages, and it emphasized how psychiatry's diagnostic vocabulary has surpassed other languages (religious, existential, moral, political) in an increasing number of contexts. This is a threat to our capabilities of seeing people's problems in social and political terms, and it risks individualizing and pathologizing the distress that people feel. Chapters 4 and 7 included references to empirical work on how adults diagnosed with ADHD use their diagnosis in processes of self-interpretation, with the diagnosis often operating in complex practices of subjectification. There is no mechanical determinism involved, such that people diagnosed will become just as the diagnosis predicts, but there are instead various looping effects at work, as Hacking has demonstrated, which means that it is hard to predict what will happen with the introduction of a new diagnosis. One must look at concrete cases and beware of formulating *a priori* conclusions.

Following Hacking, I argued in Chapter 2 that diagnoses refer to human rather than natural kinds, which means that there is an interaction between classifications and classified, mediated by numerous institutional, cultural and societal practices. So, all in all, we may conclude that there are certainly processes of pathologization, and, more broadly, psychiatrization at work in modern diagnostic cultures, but it seems unwarranted to conclude that these are always problematic for the people involved. They may certainly be problematic, but people are often capable of action and creatively interpreting and using the diagnoses they are given, so although a diagnosis may be stigmatizing and contribute to the maintenance of a problem in a person's life, it may also work to externalize the problem and provide opportunities for fruitful action for a diagnosed person. Jutel and Nettleton sum up nicely on the complexities involved: "A diagnosis can vindicate and blame, can legitimise or stigmatise, can facilitate access to resources just as it can restrict opportunities. A diagnosis can be welcomed or eschewed" (Jutel & Nettleton, 2011, p. 797)

Although I believe that we should strive for a fair and balanced assessment of the roles of psychiatric diagnoses in modern society, I do think that it is relevant to sum up some of the problems that are related to the widespread use of diagnoses. Such a list has been made by the medical sociologist Dorte Gannik, who we met in Chapter 7, with the final two problems being my own additions (adapted from Gannik, 2009):

1. No treatment may be initiated until a diagnosis has been formulated. Valuable time may thus be lost.
2. The treatment may be standardized based on the diagnostic category.
3. The diagnosis invites an either/or mode of thinking: either one gets treated or not at all.
4. Atypical and mixed conditions are not addressed or misdiagnosed.

5. This also applies to cases that lack pathological evidence.
6. The hospital sector receives a disproportionately large amount of the resources available.
7. The everyday life of the sufferer and the context of the disorder are easily ignored.
8. The intended effect of the treatment is in focus while other effects are sidelined.
9. The diagnosis individualizes a problem that may be social in nature.
10. If all you have is a hammer, everything looks like a nail – and if all you have is a diagnostic manual, everything will look like a symptom.

Some of these problems are related to overdiagnosis. Overdiagnosis happens when the diagnosis frames something that is not harmful for the diagnosed person, but which leads to harmful consequences, perhaps because a treatment is initiated with severe side-effects. I believe that future research should address the possible negative side-effects of psychiatric diagnoses themselves: it is not just psychopharmacological products that have side-effects; so can the process of being diagnosed and initiating an interpretation of one's life in light of a new diagnostic category. Although a diagnosis may be externalizing, as I have argued, it may also assist in producing a patient identity, where the person might have trouble finding developmental pathways in life other than those predicated by the deficit-oriented diagnosis. It will be worthwhile to study specifically when a diagnosis leads to improved living conditions for people and when it leads to worsened conditions, perhaps as a result of pathologization.

That a diagnosis may have unfruitful consequences is a paradox, since diagnoses are formulated with the goal of helping people. In the introduction to the book, I referred to a television show that in many ways incarnated several paradoxes (or at least contradictions) that are more generally associated with the diagnostic cultures that I have described and analyzed in this book: (1) through diagnoses, psychiatric problems are addressed as medical problems – and yet they are not just that; (2) through diagnoses, psychiatric problems are equated with manifest and sometimes transient symptoms – and yet diagnoses have a tendency to reinforce chronicity; (3) through diagnoses, psychiatric problems appear as "nothing special", because many of us could be diagnosed – and yet normalizing the disorders may cause problems for people if it means that their problems cannot be recognized as sufficiently serious. It seems clear that diagnostic cultures are inherently paradoxical.

Between Diagnostic Categories and Human Experience

I have already touched upon my answers to the next main question that I posed: that of how diagnoses are put to use by individuals who are diagnosed (or increasingly understand themselves in light of diagnostic categories). The answer was that diagnoses are used in many different ways for many different purposes, some of them existential and moral (to be able to better understand oneself and act adequately in one's life), while others are more instrumental (for obtaining welfare benefits, for instance). But the theoretical crux of the matter seems to centre on how the process of understanding oneself through the diagnosis can be spelled out: what is the relationship between diagnostic categories and human experience?

In Chapter 2 I argued that diagnoses are epistemic objects that make possible having, being, and doing mental disorders in specific ways. This is not to say that diagnostic categories uniquely determine one's experiences, but they certainly influence them. They operate as semiotic mediators, as I argued in Chapter 4, often coupled with technologies of quantification that assist in creating quantitative psychiatric subjectivities, which was one of the topics of Chapter 5. In fact, the analyses of this book emphasize that it is close to impossible to disentangle the categorical designations of suffering and distress from the experience of that same suffering and distress (see also Nielsen, 2015). This has also been argued by Tekin in a discussion of the self as involved in looping effects, following Hacking: "it is not easy – if indeed possible – to discriminate the influence of diagnosis of mental disorder on self-concepts and behavior from that of the mental disorder itself" (Tekin, 2014, p. 228).

If this is so, we should in future research address the interrelationships between experiences of distress and the categories we invoke to describe and understand that distress. In psychology there is a conventional distinction between sensations (raw, uninterpreted feelings), perceptions (when the feelings are interpreted as feelings of something), and cognitions (the conscious and reflective understanding of something through the use of rational categories). In relation to our themes in this book, this distinction would lead to an awareness of how *sensory markers* (unpleasant experiences, corresponding to sensations in psychology) lead to *symptoms* (corresponding to perceptions), and finally, if there is a sufficient number of symptoms, to *diagnoses* (corresponding to cognitions). The arrows of influence should point in both directions at the same time, since we know that more reflective understandings and categories may influence how we perceive and experience something. There is an extremely complex interplay of sensory experiences (of fatigue, hyperactivity etc.), symptoms, and diagnoses, each being capable of influencing the others. This is what cultural psychology with its emphasis on semiotic mediation, and its further perspective on relations to larger social practices and societal structures is capable of addressing. It may happen on large, macro sociological scales, as I argued in Chapter 5, where the logic of quantification has become inscribed in numerous societal practices, including those that deal with human problems.

This book's approach to mental disorder should lead us to be suspicious of theories that point to discrete and isolated causes behind people's problems. As Bolton concludes (and many other scholars cited in this book would agree): "no (practically no) psychiatric conditions have a single, specific cause" (Bolton, 2008, p. 5). Recognizing this, as I argued in Chapter 2, should lead us to give up essentialist, natural kind understandings of mental disorder. Instead, we should focus on developing relational and situational models, such as the one I suggested in Chapter 7. That was a cultural psychological theory (aided by Gannik and Mol) that focused on normativity and on the interplay of various forces or mediators stemming from the brain, the body, social practices (with their norms and discursive categories) and also technologies and artefacts. Mental disorders emerge as *persons'* problems (and not, for example, as the problems of brains) amidst these different forces and mediators, and future applied research should study how to develop supportive resources across these sets of mediators to help people with their problems. Sometimes this may involve "changing the person" (the brain or the person's self-interpretations), sometimes it may involve changing environmental conditions or artefacts, and sometimes it may involve changing the discursive categorizations, which may themselves contribute to the creation of suffering. What should be made clear is that although the current diagnostic understanding of people's problems is flawed, and although there are probably massive processes of pathologization taking place, this should not lead us to argue in favour of withholding help from people. As Joan Busfield has put it:

> To argue that problems [...] are not mental illnesses is not to contend that those with such problems should not seek help for them, or that help should not be provided. It is to argue that it is not helpful to pathologize such difficulties, since viewing them as mental illnesses locates the problem within the person. It leads to efforts to change individuals, often by prescribing psychoactive medications, or encouraging them to change the way they think about their experiences, rather than seeing the problems as lying within the features of society in which they live. (Busfield, 2011, p. 195)

Recently, Alastair Morgan has asked if psychiatry is dying (Morgan, 2015). Like many analysts in this book, he concludes that the idea "that there are discrete mental illnesses with clear boundaries that we should endeavor to codify and classify and utilise to validate aetiologically is no longer a useful way of structuring a response to mental distress" (Morgan, 2015, p. 157). He lists five critical positions that play a role in the current crisis of psychiatry, which is comparable to that of the 20th century which led to the anti-psychiatric movement. The positions are:

(1) Cognitive/behavioural neuroscience, which wants to leave the symptom-based approach and develop psychiatry in a biological direction. The recent initiative by the U.S. National Institute of Mental Health (directed by Thomas Insel) to concentrate on Research Domain Criteria (RDoC) is the most visible example. However, this could easily lead to psychiatry becoming a branch of biology (instead of medicine) and thus have reductionist consequences. Against this, I have argued in this book that we need to maintain that *persons* (and not their brains) are the subjects of mental disorder.

(2) Poststructuralism, which is represented most clearly by Nikolas Rose, who has studied how subjectivity appears today through the biomedical sciences

and how we therefore become neurochemical selves (Rose, 2003). This is a posthumanist turn that is descriptive rather than critical.

(3) Conservative pluralism, represented by figures such as Allan Frances, who criticize the expansion of psychiatry and its categories and call for better diagnostics that are able to "save the normal" from pathologization.

(4) Critical psychiatry, which emphasizes recovery and criticizes mainstream psychiatry for neglecting the social contexts of suffering and the subjective meanings that people attach to their problems.

(5) Radical pluralism, which, for Morgan, represents an attempt to revive psychoanalytic and deep phenomenological ideas. It is not so much that mental illness is a myth, as some of the critical psychiatrists say (following in the footsteps of Szasz), but rather that mental health is a myth, because – to paraphrase Freud – life is characterized by "common misery" ("*allgemeines Elend*").

We may conclude that the relational-situational approach to mental disorder and diagnoses, represented by cultural psychology, has something in common with each of these perspectives (all of which contain something valuable, according to Morgan). With the first perspective, it shares an interest in the brain – not, however, conceived as an agent or locus of mental disorder, but as a significant tool in the life projects of persons, and a tool that may be broken relative to the norms and concerns of social practices. With the second, it shares an interest in how subjectivity is affected by the categories and technologies of modern society, although it does not posit a determinism of interpellation (according to which subjectivity is a mere epiphenomenon of discursive practices), but instead puts the acting person centre-stage. With the third perspective, it shares a concern that current psychiatry pathologizes far too many human conditions, and with the fourth and fifth, it takes an interest in the experiences of suffering people, which should be the starting point for scientific explorations into human problems and for developing humane ways of addressing these problems.

Like few other theories, the cultural psychological approach, as I have invoked it in this book, is able to integrate various complementary strands, in particular a phenomenological strand (emphasizing human experience in intentional worlds), a semiotic-discursive strand (emphasizing semiotic mediation), and finally an object oriented strand (focusing on the role of technology and artefact mediation in human cultural life) (see Figure 1.1 in Chapter 1). All three angles are necessary if one wishes to understand mental disorder as fully as possible, and I am certain that future research ought to strive for pluralism rather than seek monolithic theoretical answers to something as complex and many-sided as human suffering and distress.

Diagnostic Cultures in Societal Perspective

The book has not only charted contemporary diagnostic cultures, but it has also related the emergence of these to underlying societal developments. I have referred to Bauman's notion of liquid modernity (in Chapters 5 and 6) and also to other sociological diagnoses of our times, and this is relevant when seeking to answer the question: how do personal problems interact with broader societal trends, and how can this be studied? In order to answer this, I wish to return to my main example of ADHD and provide a comparative reading of this disorder and depression (which I have also referred to a number of times), as this reading may shed light on current societal norms of personhood. The person with ADHD and the person with depression exemplify opposite ways of diverging from these norms. (What follows is inspired by Petersen & Brinkmann, 2015.)

The ideal self today (in our liquid modern world) is an enterprising self that is active, creative and positive. The ideal self relates to itself as a reservoir of competencies that are to be monitored and developed. This involves a curious mix of self-control (being able to constantly work and optimize oneself) and self-transgression (being constantly on the move, and engaged in lifelong learning in learning organizations). Two of the most prevalent "epidemics" of mental disorder are depression and ADHD. Both are treated with psychopharmaceuticals, and both have been on the rise in many Western countries during the last couple of decades. They are also different, of course, as depression is more often diagnosed among women (and adults) and ADHD is more often diagnosed among men (and children), although this might be changing toward a more equal distribution. But what interests me here are the differences in symptomatology: depression is characterized by a feeling of impotence and weariness, by an experience of not being able to catch up and perform, and notably by anhedonia or a lack of desire. The depressed person does not really desire anything and is not able to see that her situation might change in the future (Rønberg, 2014). She is oriented toward the past, about which she worries and ruminates, and not toward developing into the future. The depressed person is slow and sad.

This is in contrast to the person with ADHD, who is too fast in a sense, sometimes even close to manic. The person with ADHD lives too much in the future and too little in the past. She is constantly ahead of herself, having difficulties maintaining a presence in the here and now. Unlike the depressed person with a diminished level of activity, the person with ADHD has a heightened level – she is *hyper*active. Whereas the depressed person thinks too much without being able to act, the person with ADHD acts too much, in a sense, without being able to hold a thought. Depression is a social pathology in a liquid modern world that demands self-transgression, for the depressed person is unable to transgress. ADHD becomes a social pathology in a liquid modern world that demands self-control, for this is a challenge for the hyperactive person in a culture with few external limits (as the person must impose the limits herself, which presupposes self-control).

I end this book with this short reading of the disorders of depression and ADHD as two opposed ways of being "wrong" relative to societal demands. The big question thus becomes: are people with these disorders thus really ill, or are they simply pathologized because of societal demands and practices? This question was addressed in Chapter 6, which presented a number of interpretations of the epidemics of mental disorders today. In one way, this question turns out to be somewhat scholastic, with few practical consequences, and the proper approach to it – in light of this book's views on the entanglements of cultural, biological and social forces that generate what we call mental disorder (cf. the fourth question posed above) – is to point to the doubled-edged process in modern diagnostic cultures: our fluidly modern world is likely to generate new forms of suffering (based on the experience of not being able to catch up and/or control oneself) *and* these forms of suffering are increasingly interpreted in diagnostic terms, since the diagnostic language of suffering has become the default position. These are the two sides of the diagnostic cultures that researchers need to keep interrogating in future research, and we need to enlarge our awareness of what generates human suffering to encompass much more than what can be understood through the diagnostic manuals. We need a theoretical account that is able to include factors as varied as the brain and societal structures. This presupposes a willingness on behalf of researchers to communicate across existing disciplinary divides: neuroscientists should discuss with sociologists and vice versa; psychologists should study the work of anthropologists and vice versa. This seems to be the only way forward in a time of crises for psychiatry.

References

Aarhus Kommune (2013). *ADHD-strategi for voksne i Social og Beskæftigelsesforvaltningen.*

Abraham, J. (2010). Pharmaceuticalization of society in context: Theoretical, empirical and health dimensions. *Sociology*, 44, 603–622.

Adler, L.A. & Shaw, D. (2011). Diagnosis ADHD in adults. In J. Buitelaar, C. Kan, & P. Asherson (Eds), *ADHD in Adults: Characterization, Diagnosis, and Treatment.* Cambridge: Cambridge University Press.

Angel, K. (2012). Contested psychiatric ontology and feminist critique: 'Female sexual dysfunction' and the Diagnostic and Statistical Manual. *History of the Human Sciences*, 25, 3–24.

Armstrong, D. (1995). The rise of surveillance medicine. *Sociology of Health & Illness*, 17, 393–404.

Barkley, R. (1997). *ADHD and the Nature of Self-Control.* New York: Guilford Press.

Baroncelli, L. (2015). *Depression and 'crises of meaninglessness' in the political-economic theology of the money-God.* (Unpublished doctoral thesis). Cork: Department of Sociology. National University of Ireland.

Barsky, A. (1988). The paradox of health. *New England Journal of Medicine*, 318, 414–418.

Bauman, Z. (2007). *Consuming Life.* Cambridge: Polity Press.

Bennett, M.R. & Hacker, P.M.S. (2003). *Philosophical Foundations of Neuroscience.* Oxford: Blackwell.

Billig, M. (1999). *Freudian Repression: Conversation Creating the Unconscious.* Cambridge: Cambridge University Press.

Bolton, D. (2008). *What is Mental Disorder? An Essay in Philosophy, Science, and Values.* Oxford: Oxford University Press.

Bolton, D. (2010). Conceptualisation of mental disorder and its personal meanings. *Journal of Mental Health*, 19, 328–336.

Boorse, C. (1976). What a theory of mental health should be. *Journal for the Theory of Social Behaviour*, 6, 61–84.

Bowden, G. (2014). The merit of sociological accounts of disorder: The Attention-Deficit Hyperactivity Disorder case. *Health*, 18, 422–438.

Bowker, G.C. & Star, S.L. (2000). *Sorting Things Out: Classification and Its Consequences.* Cambridge, MA: The MIT Press.

Boyle, M. (2011). Making the world go away, and how psychology and psychiatry benefit. In M. Rapley, J. Moncrieff, & J. Dillon (Eds), *De-Medicalizing Misery:*

Psychiatry, Psychology and the Human Condition Basingstoke: Palgrave Macmillan, pp. 27–43.

Brinkmann, S. (2005). Human kinds and looping effects in psychology: Foucauldian and hermeneutic perspectives. *Theory & Psychology*, 15, 769–791.

Brinkmann, S. (2006). Mental life in the space of reasons. *Journal for the Theory of Social Behaviour*, 36, 1–16.

Brinkmann, S. (2008). Identity as self-interpretation. *Theory & Psychology*, 18, 404–422.

Brinkmann, S. (2011a). *Psychology as a Moral Science: Perspectives on Normativity*. New York: Springer.

Brinkmann, S. (2011b). Towards an expansive hybrid psychology: Integrating theories of the mediated mind. *Integrative Psychological and Behavioral Science*, 45, 1–20.

Brinkmann, S. (2012). The mind as skills and dispositions: On normativity and mediation. *Integrative Psychological and Behavioral Science*, 46, 78–89.

Brinkmann, S. (2013a). *John Dewey: Science for a Changing World*. New Brunswick, NJ: Transaction Publishers.

Brinkmann, S. (2013b). The pathologization of morality. In K. Keohane & A. Petersen (Eds), *The Social Pathologies of Contemporary Civilization* Farnham: Ashgate, pp. 103–118.

Brinkmann, S. (2014a). Languages of suffering. *Theory & Psychology*, 24, 630–648.

Brinkmann, S. (2014b). Psychiatric diagnoses as semiotic mediators: The case of ADHD. *Nordic Psychology*, 66, 121–134.

Brown, T. (2005). *Attention Deficit Disorder: The Unfocused Mind in Children and Adults*. New Haven: Yale University Press.

Buitelaar, J., Kan, C.C., & Asherson, P. (2011). *ADHD in Adults: Characterization, Diagnosis, and Treatment*. Cambridge: Cambridge University Press.

Busfield, J. (2011). *Mental Illness*. Cambridge: Polity.

Charland, L.C. (2004). Character: Moral Treatment and the Personality Disorders. In J. Radden (Ed.), *The Philosophy of Psychiatry: A Companion*. Oxford: Oxford University Press.

Church, J. (2004). Social constructionist models: Making order out of disorder – On the social construction of madness. In J. Radden (Ed.), *The Philosophy of Psychiatry* Oxford: Oxford University Press, pp. 393–406.

Clarke, A. & Shim, J. (2010). Medicalization and biomedicalization revisited: Technoscience and transformations of health, illness and American medicine. In B.A. Pescosolido, J.K. Martin, J.D. McLeod, & A. Rogers (Eds), *Handbook of the Sociology of Health, Illness, and Healing*. New York: Springer, pp. 173–199.

Cole, M. (2003). *Kulturpsykologi*. København: Hans Reitzels Forlag.

Collin, F. (1990). Naturlige klasser, semantik og metode i samfundsvidenskaberne. *Filosofiske studier*, 11, 7–24.

Comstock, E.J. (2011). The end of drugging children: Toward the genealogy of the ADHD subject. *Journal of the History of the Behavioral Sciences*, 47, 44–69.

Conrad, P. (2006). *Identifying Hyperactive Children: The Medicalization of Deviant Behavior*. (2nd expanded edition). Aldershot: Ashgate.

Conrad, P. (2007). *The Medicalization of Society*. Baltimore: The Johns Hopkins University Press.

Cooper, R. (2014). *Diagnosing the Diagnostic and Statistical Manual of Mental Disorders*. London: Karnac.

Coulter, J. (1979). *The Social Construction of Mind: Studies in Ethnomethodology and Linguistic Philosophy*. London: Macmillan.

Danziger, K. (1990). *Constructing the Subject: Historical Origins of Psychological Research*. Cambridge: Cambridge University Press.

Danziger, K. (1996). The practice of psychological discourse. In C.F. Graumann & K.J. Gergen (Eds), *Historical Dimensions of Psychological Discourse*. Cambridge: Cambridge University Press.

Danziger, K. (1997). *Naming the Mind: How Psychology Found Its Language*. London: Sage.

Danziger, K. (1999). Natural Kinds, Human Kinds, and Historicity. In W. Maiers, B. Bayer, B. Duarte Esgalhado, R. Jorna, & E. Schraube (Eds), *Challenges to Theoretical Psychology*. North York, Ontario: Captus Press.

Danziger, K. (2003). Where history, theory, and philosophy meet: The biography of psychological objects. In D.B. Hill & M.J. Kral (Eds), *About Psychology: Essays at the Crossroads of History, Theory, and Philosophy*. Albany, NY: State University of New York Press.

Daston, L. & Galison, P. (2007). *Objectivity*. New York: Zone Books.

Ebeling, M. (2011). 'Get with the program!': Pharmaceutical marketing, symptom checklists and self-diagnosis. *Social Science & Medicine*, 73, 825–832.

Faraone, S.V. & Biederman, J. (2005). What is the prevalence of adult ADHD? Results of a population screen of 966 adults. *Journal of Attention Disorders*, 9, 384–391.

Foucault, M. (1988). Technologies of the Self. In *Technologies of the Self*. London: Tavistock Publications.

Foucault, M. (1994). The Subject and Power. In J.D. Faubion (Ed.), *Power: Essential Works of Michel Foucault, Vol. 3*. London: Penguin.

Frances, A. (2013). *Saving Normal*. New York: HarperCollins.

Fuchs, T. (2009). Embodied cognitive neuroscience and its consequences for psychiatry. *Poiesis & Praxis*, 6, 219–233.

Furedi, F. (2004). *Therapy Culture: Cultivating Vulnerability in an Uncertain Age*. London: Routledge.

Furedi, F. (2008). Medicalisation in a therapy culture. In D. Wainwright (Ed.), *A Sociology of Health*. London: Sage, pp. 97–115.

Gannik, D. (2005). *Social sygdomsteori: Et situationelt perspektiv*. Frederiksberg: Samfundslitteratur.

Gannik, D. (2009). Diagnosen som sygdomskonstruktion: Er der et alternativ? *Månedsskrift for Praktisk Lægegerning*, 87, 1284–1292.

Gee, J.P. (2005). *An Introduction to Discourse Analysis: Theory and Method.* London: Routledge.

Gergen, K. (1994). *Realities and Relationships.* Cambridge, MA: Harvard University Press.

Giddens, A. (1976). *New Rules of Sociological Method.* London: Hutchinson.

Gigerenzer, G. (1996). From tools to theories: Discovery in cognitive psychology. In C.F. Graumann & K.J. Gergen (Eds), *Historical Dimensions of Psychological Discourse.* Cambridge: Cambridge University Press.

Gillespie, A., Best, C., & O'Neill, B. (2012). Cognitive function and assistive technology for cognition: A systematic review. *Journal of the International Neuropsychological Society*, 18, 1–19.

Gillespie, A. & Zittoun, T. (2010). Using resources: Conceptualizing the mediation and reflective use of tools and signs. *Culture & Psychology*, 16, 37–62.

Goffman, E. (1961). *Asylums.* New York: Doubleday.

Hacking, I. (1986). Making Up People. In T.C. Heller, M. Sosna, & D. Wellbery (Eds), *Reconstructing Individualism.* Stanford: Stanford University Press.

Hacking, I. (1990). *The Taming of Chance.* Cambridge: Cambridge University Press.

Hacking, I. (1995a). *Rewriting the Soul.* Princeton, NJ: Princeton University Press.

Hacking, I. (1995b). The Looping Effect of Human Kinds. In D. Sperber, D. Premack, & A.J. Premack (Eds), *Causal Cognition: A Multidisciplinary Debate.* Oxford: Clarendon Press.

Hacking, I. (1998). *Mad Travelers: Reflections on the Reality of Transient Mental Disease.* Charlottesville: University Press of Virginia.

Hacking, I. (2006). Kinds of People: Moving Targets. *British Academy Lecture*, 11 April 2006 (web version).

Halleröd, S.L.H., Anckarsäter, H., Råstam, M., & Scherman, M.H. (2015). Experienced consequences of being diagnosed with ADHD as an adult – a qualitative study. *BMC Psychiatry*, 15, 1–13.

Harré, R. (1983). *Personal Being.* Oxford: Basil Blackwell.

Harré, R. (2002). *Cognitive Science: A Philosophical Introduction.* London: Sage.

Harré, R. & Moghaddam, F.M. (2012). *Psychology for the Third Millennium: Integrating Cultural and Neuroscience Perspectives.* Thousand Oaks, CA: Sage.

Harré, R., Moghaddam, F.M., Cairnie, T.P., Rothbart, D., & Sabat, S. (2009). Recent advances in positioning theory. *Theory & Psychology*, 19, 5–31.

Haslam, N.O. (1998). Natural Kinds, Human Kinds, and Essentialism. *Social Research*, 65, 291–315.

Haslam, N.O. (2014). Natural kinds in psychiatry: Conceptually implausible, empirically questionable, and stigmatizing. In H. Kincaid & J. Sullivan (Eds), *Classifying Psychopathology: Mental Kinds and Natural Kinds.* Cambridge, MA: The MIT Press.

Healy, D. (2012). *Pharmageddon*. Berkeley, CA: University of California Press.

Hegel, G.W.F. (1821). *Elements of the Philosophy of Right*. (1991 Edition). Cambridge: Cambridge University Press.

Heidegger, M. (1927). *Being and Time*. (1962 Edition). New York: HarperCollins Publishers.

Hermann, S. & Kristensen, J.E. (2005). Fra strejke til stress. *Information*, 12–05–2005.

Hollis, M. (1977). *Models of Man: Philosophical Thoughts on Social Action*. Cambridge: Cambridge University Press.

Honneth, A. (2004). Organized Self-Realization. *European Journal of Social Theory*, 7, 463–478.

Honneth, A. (2008). *Reification: A New Look at an Old Idea*. Oxford: Oxford University Press.

Horwitz, A.V. (2002). *Creating Mental Illness*. Chicago: University of Chicago Press.

Horwitz, A.V. (2010). Pharmaceuticals and the medicalization of social life. In D.W. Light (Ed.), *The Risks of Prescription Drugs*. New York: Columbia University Press.

Horwitz, A.V. & Wakefield, J.C. (2005). The Age of Depression. *The Public Interest*, 158, 39–58.

Horwitz, A.V. & Wakefield, J.C. (2007). *The Loss of Sadness: How Psychiatry Transformed Normal Sorrow into Depressive Disorder*. Oxford: Oxford University Press.

Horwitz, A.V. & Wakefield, J.C. (2012). *All We Have to Fear: Psychiatry's Transformation of Natural Anxieties into Mental Disorders*. Oxford: Oxford University Press.

Husserl, E. (1954). *Die Krisis der europäischen Wissenschaften und die tranzendentale Phänomenologie*. Haag: Martinus Nijhoff.

Illouz, E. (2007). *Cold Intimacies: The Making of Emotional Capitalism*. Cambridge: Polity Press.

Ingold, T. (2011). *Being Alive: Essays on Movement, Knowledge and Description*. London: Routledge.

Jaspers, K. (1997). *General Psychopathology*. (First published 1959). Baltimore, MA: The Johns Hopkins University Press.

Jensen, A.F. (2009). *Projektsamfundet*. Aarhus: Aarhus University Press.

Jensen, V.S. (2015). What are we talking about when we talk about autism? Exploring a layered account approach. *Departures in Critical Qualitative Research*, Forthcoming.

Joseph, J. (2009). ADHD and genetics: A consensus reconsidered. In S. Timimi & J. Leo (Eds), *Rethinking ADHD: From Brain to Culture*. Basingstoke: Palgrave Macmillan, pp. 58–91.

Jutel, A.G. (2011). *Putting a Name to It: Diagnosis in Contemporary Society*. Baltimore: The Johns Hopkins University Press.

Jutel, A.G. & Nettleton, S. (2011). Toward a sociology of diagnosis: Reflections and opportunities. *Social Science & Medicine*, 73, 793–800.

Keohane, K. & Petersen, A. (2013). *The Social Pathologies of Contemporary Civilization*. Farnham: Ashgate.

Kessler, R.C. (2010). The prevalence of mental illness. In T. Scheid & T.N. Brown (Eds), *A Handbook for the Study of Mental Health: Social Contexts, Theories, and Systems* (2nd edition). Cambridge: Cambridge University Press, pp. 46–63.

Kierkegaard, S.A. (1844). *The Concept of Anxiety*. (1981 Edition). Princeton, NJ: Princeton University Press.

Kierkegaard, S.A. (1995). *Sygdommen til Døden*. (First published 1849). Copenhagen: Gyldendals bogklubber.

Kilgus, M.D. & Rea, W.S. (2014). Introduction: Clinical decision making. In M.D. Kilgus & W.S. Rea (Eds), *Essential Psychopathology Casebook*. New York: W.W. Norton & Co., pp. 1–12.

Kincaid, H. & Sullivan, J. (2014). Classifying psychopathology: Mental kinds and natural kinds. In H. Kincaid & J. Sullivan (Eds), *Classifying Psychopathology: Mental Kinds and Natural Kinds*. Cambridge, MA: The MIT Press, pp. 1–10.

Kirkegaard, T. & Brinkmann, S. (2015). Rewriting stress: Toward a cultural psychology of collective stress at work. *Culture & Psychology*, 21, 81–94.

Kofod, E.H. (2013). Grief: From morality to pathology. In preparation.

Kofod, E.H. (2015). Grief as a border diagnosis. In press.

Kohn, R., Saxena, S., Levav, I., & Saraceno, B. (2004). The treatment gap in mental health care. *Bulletin of the World Health Organization*, 82, 858–866.

Kutchins, H. & Kirk, S. (1997). *Making Us Crazy – DSM: The Psychiatric Bible and the Creation of Mental Disorders*. Chicago: University of Chicago Press.

Kyhn, D.B. (2012). *Gal eller normal: Fortællinger om psykisk sygdom*. København: Lindhardt & Ringhof.

Lane, C. (2007). *Shyness: How Normal Behavior Became a Sickness*. New Haven: Yale University Press.

Latour, B. (2005). *Reassembling the Social*. Oxford: Oxford University Press.

Lauveng, A. (2008). *I morgen var jeg altid en løve*. København: Akademisk Forlag.

Lazarus, R. & Folkman, S. (1984). *Stress, Appraisal and Coping*. New York: Springer.

Lilienfield, S.O. & Marino, L. (1995). Mental disorder as a Roschian concept: A crtitique of Wakefield's 'harmful dysfunction' analysis. *Journal of Abnormal Psychology*, 104, 411–420.

Lilleleht, E. (2003). Progress and Power: Exploring the Disciplinary Connections between Moral Treatment and Psychiatric Rehabilitation. *Philosophy, Psychiatry & Psychology*, 9, 167–182.

Littlewood, R. (2002). *Pathologies of the West: An Anthropology of Mental Illness in Europe and America*. Ithaca, NY: Cornell University Press.

Lock, M. (2001). The tempering of medical anthropology: Troubling natural categories. *Medical Anthropology Quarterly*, 15, 478–492.

Lock, M. & Nguyen, V.K. (2010). *An Anthropology of Biomedicine*. Chichester, UK: Wiley-Blackwell.

Lupton, D. & Jutel, A.G. (2015). 'It's like having a physician in your pocket!' A critical analysis of self-diagnosis smartphone appls. *Social Science & Medicine*, 133, 128–135.

MacIntyre, A. (1999). *Dependent Rational Animals – Why Human Beings Need the Virtues*. London: Duckworth.

Maiese, M. (2012). Rethinking attention deficit hyperactivity disorder. *Philosophical Psychology*, 25, 893–916.

Martin, E. (2007). *Bipolar Expeditions: Mania and Depression in American Culture*. Princeton, NJ: Princeton University Press.

Martin, J. & Sugarman, J. (2001). Interpreting human kinds: Beginnings of a hermeneutic psychology. *Theory & Psychology*, 11, 193–207.

Marx, K. (1971). *Capital*. (Vol. III). London: Lawrence and Wishart.

Maser, J.D. & Gallup, G.G. (1990). Theism as a by-product of natural selection. *Journal of Religion*, 70, 71–83.

McDowell, J. (1994). *Mind and World*. Cambridge, MA: Harvard University Press.

McGann, P. J. (2011). Troubling diagnoses. In P.J. McGann & D.J. Hutson (Eds), *Sociology of Diagnosis*. Bingley, UK: Emerald, pp. 331–362.

McLennan, G. (2010). The postsecular turn. *Theory, Culture & Society*, 27, 3–20.

Mills, C.W. (1959). *The Sociological Imagination*. (2000 Edition). Oxford: Oxford University Press.

Mol, A. (2002). *The Body Multiple: Ontology in Medical Practice*. Durham, NC: Duke University Press.

Morgan, A. (2014). The happiness turn: Axel Honneth, self-reification and 'sickness unto health'. *Subjectivity*, 7, 219–233.

Morgan, A. (2015). Is psychiatry dying? Crisis and critique in contemporary psychiatry. *Social Theory & Health*, 13, 141–161.

Moynihan, R. & Cassels, A. (2005). *Selling Sickness: How the worlds biggest drug companies are turning us all into patients*. New York: Nation Books.

Murphy, J.M., Laird, N.M., Monson, R.R., Sobol, A.M., & Leighton, A.H. (2000). A 40-year perspective on the prevalence of depression: The Stirling County Study. *Archives of General Psychiatry*, 57, 209–215.

Musaeus, P. & Brinkmann, S. (2011). The semiosis of family conflict: A case study of home-based psychotherapy. *Culture & Psychology*, 17, 47–63.

Nielsen, M. (2015). Becoming ADHD. In preparation.

Nielsen, M. & Grøn, L. (2013). Quantify your self! Numbers in ambiguous borderlands of health. *Tidsskrift for Forskning i Sygdom og Samfund*, 19, 55–74.

Nordahl, T., Sunnevåg, A.-K., Aasen, A.M., & Kostøl, A. (2010). *Uligheder og variationer: Rapport til skolens rejsehold*. Aalborg: University College Nordjylland.

Parsons, T. (1975). The sick role and the role of the physician reconsidered. *The Milbank Memorial Fund Quarterly. Health and Society*, 53, 257–278.

Paterson, M. (2006). *Consumption and Everyday Life*. London: Routledge.

Petersen, A. (2011). Authentic self-realization and depression. *International Sociology*, 26, 5–24.

Petersen, A. & Brinkmann, S. (2015). Diagnosekultur: Sociale patologier og kulturanalyse. In P.T. Andersen & M.H. Jacobsen (Eds), *Kultursociologi og kulturanalyse*. København: Hans Reitzels Forlag.

Pickersgill, M. (2012). What is psychiatry? Co-producing complexity in mental health. *Social Theory & Health*, 10, 328–347.

Progler, Y. (2009). Mental illness and social stigma: Notes on "How mad are you?". *Journal of Research in Medical Sciences*, 14, 331–334.

Putnam, H. (1973). Meaning and Reference. *The Journal of Philosophy*, 70, 699–711.

Putnam, H. (1999). *The Threefold Cord: Mind, Body, and World*. New York: Columbia University Press.

Richards, G. (1996). *Putting Psychology in Its Place: An Introduction from a Critical Historical Perspective*. London: Routledge.

Rimke, H. & Hunt, A. (2002). From sinners to degenerates: the medicaliztion of morality in the 19th century. *History of the Human Sciences*, 15, 59–88.

Ringer, A. (2013). *Listening to patients: A study of illness discourses, patient identity, and user involvement in contemporary psychiatric practice*. Roskilde University: PhD Dissertation.

Robinson, D.N. (1996). *Wild Beasts and Idle Humours: The Insanity Defense from Antiquity to the Present*. Cambridge, MA: Harvard University Press.

Robinson, D.N. (2002). *Praise and Blame: Moral Realism and its Applications*. Princeton, NJ: Princeton University Press.

Rønberg, M. (2014). The lack of future in depression. In preparation.

Rønberg, M. (2015). Struggling with depression: Individual negotiations with diagnostic categories. Submitted.

Rorty, R. (1979). *Philosophy and the Mirror of Nature*. Princeton, NJ: Princeton University Press.

Rosa, H. (2003). Social Acceleration: Ethical and Political Consequences of a Desynchronized High-Speed Society. *Constellations*, 10, 3–33.

Rose, N. (1996). Power and subjectivity: Critical history and psychology. In C.F. Graumann & K.J. Gergen (Eds), *Historical Dimensions of Psychological Discourse*. Cambridge: Cambridge University Press.

Rose, N. (1999). *Governing the Soul: The Shaping of the Private Self*. (2nd. ed.). London: Free Association Books.

Rose, N. (2003). Neurochemical Selves. *Society*, 41, 46–59.

Rose, N. (2006). Disorders without borders? The expanding scope of psychiatric practice. *BioSocieties*, 1, 465–484.

Rose, N. (2007). *The Politics of Life Itself: Biomedicine, Power and Subjectivity in the Twenty-First Century*. Princeton, NJ: Princeton University Press.

Rose, N. (2013). *What is diagnosis for?* Talk given at the Institute of Psychiatry, King's College, London: Retrieved from: http://nikolasrose.com/wp-content/uploads/2013/07/Rose-2013-What-is-diagnosis-for-IoP-revised-July-2013.pdf.

Rose, N. & Abi-Rached, J.M. (2013). *Neuro: The New Brain Sciences and the Management of the Mind.* Princeton, NJ: Princeton University Press.

Rosenberg, C.E. (2007). *Our Present Complaint: American Medicine, Then and Now.* Baltimore: The Johns Hopkins University Press.

Schmitz, M.F., Filippone, P., & Edelman, E.M. (2003). Social representations of Attention Deficit/Hyperactivity Disorder, 1988–1997. *Culture & Psychology*, 9, 383–406.

Schwartz, B. (2004). The tyranny of choice. *Scientific American*, 290, 70–75.

Sennett, R. (1998). *The Corrosion of Character.* New York: Norton.

Shweder, R.A. (1990). Cultural Psychology – What Is It? In J.W. Stigler, R.A. Shweder, & G. Herdt (Eds), *Cultural Psychology: Essays on Comparative Human Development.* Cambridge: Cambridge University Press.

Shweder, R.A. (2008). The cultural psychology of suffering: The many meanings of health in Orissa, India (and elsewhere). *Ethos*, 36, 60–77.

Shweder, R.A., Much, N., Mahapatra, M., & Park, L. (1997). The "Big Three" of Morality (Autonomy, Community, Divinity) and the "Big Three" Explanations of Suffering. In A.M. Brandt & P. Rozin (Eds), *Morality and Health.* London: Routledge.

Singh, I. (2011). A disorder of anger and aggression: Children's perspectives on attention deficit/hyperactivity disorder in the UK. *Social Science & Medicine*, 73, 889–896.

Singh, I. & Rose, N. (2009). Biomarkers in psychiatry. *Nature*, 460, 202–207.

Smail, D. (2011). Psychotherapy: Illusion with no future? In M. Rapley, J. Moncrieff, & J. Dillon (Eds), *De-Medicalizing Misery: Psychiatry, Psychology and the Human Condition.* Basingstoke: Palgrave Macmillan.

Smith, M. (2012). *Hyperactive: The Controversial History of ADHD.* London: Reaktion Books.

Smith, N.H. (2002). *Charles Taylor: Meaning, Morals and Modernity.* Cambridge: Polity Press.

Smith, R. (1997). *The Norton History of the Human Sciences.* New York: W.W. Norton & Co.

Sprague, E. (1999). *Persons and Their Minds.* Boulder, CO: Westview.

Sterelny, K. (2012). *The Evolved Apprentice: How Evolution Made Humans Unique.* Cambridge, MA: The MIT Press.

Strathern, M. (2000). *Audit Cultures.* London: Routledge.

Szasz, T. (1961). *The Myth of Mental Illness: Foundations of a Theory of Personal Conduct.* New York: HarperCollins.

Taylor, C. (1981). Understanding and Explanation in the *Geisteswissenschaften*. In S.M. Holtzman & C.M. Leich (Eds), *Wittgenstein: To Follow a Rule.* London: Routledge & Kegan Paul.

Taylor, C. (1985). What is human agency? In *Human Agency and Language: Philosophical Papers 1*. Cambridge: Cambridge University Press.

Taylor, C. (1989). *Sources of the Self*. Cambridge: Cambridge University Press.

Taylor, C. (1991). *The Ethics of Authenticity*. Cambridge, MA: Harvard University Press.

Taylor, C. (1999). Two Theories of Modernity. *Public Culture*, 11, 153–174.

Taylor, C. (2004). *Modern Social Imaginaries*. Durham, NC: Duke University Press.

Taylor, C. (2007). *A Secular Age*. Cambridge, MA: Harvard University Press.

Tekin, S. (2014). The missing self in Hacking's looping effects. In H. Kincaid & J. Sullivan (Eds), *Classifying Psychopathology: Mental Kinds and Natural Kinds*. Cambridge, MA: The MIT Press.

Timimi, S. (2009). Why diagnosis of ADHD has increased so rapidly in the West: A cultural perspective. In S. Timimi & J. Leo (Eds), *Rethinking ADHD: From Brain to Culture*. Basingstoke: Palgrave Macmillan, pp. 133–159.

Turner, B.S. (1991). *Religion and Social Theory*. (2nd edition). London: Sage.

Valsiner, J. (2007). *Culture in Minds and Societies: Foundations of Cultural Psychology*. New Delhi: Sage.

Valsiner, J. (2014). *An Invitation to Cultural Psychology*. London: Sage.

Valsiner, J. & Rosa, A. (2007). *The Cambridge Handbook of Sociocultural Psychology*. Cambridge: Cambridge University Press.

Valsiner, J. & van der Veer, R. (2000). *The Social Mind: Construction of the Idea*. Cambridge: Cambridge University Press.

Vygotsky, L.S. (1929). *Collected Works of L.S. Vygotsky. Volume 2: The Fundamentals of Defectology*. (1993 Edition). New York: Plenum Press.

Vygotsky, L.S. (1978). *Mind in Society: The Development of Higher Psychological Processes*. Cambridge, MA: Harvard University Press.

Wainwright, D. & Calnan, M. (2002). *Work Stress: The Making of a Modern Epidemic*. Buckingham: Open University Press.

Wakefield, J.C. (1992). The concept of mental disorder: On the boundary between biological facts and social values. *American Psychologist*, 47, 373–388.

Wakefield, J.C. (2010). Misdiagnosing normality: Psychiatry's failure to address the problem of false positive diagnoses of mental disorder in a changing professional environment. *Journal of Mental Health*, 19, 337–351.

Watters, E. (2010). *Crazy Like Us: The Globalization of the American Psyche*. New York: The Free Press.

Whitaker, R. (2010). *Anatomy of an Epidemic: Magic Bullets, Psychiatric Drugs, and the Astonishing Rise of Mental Illness in America*. New York: Broadway Paperbacks.

White, M. (2007). *Maps of Narrative Practice*. New York: W.W. Norton.

Wilkinson, I. (2005). *Suffering: A Sociological Introduction*. Cambridge: Polity Press.

Williams, R.F.G. (2009). Everyday sorrows are not mental disorders: The clash between psychiatry and Western cultural habits. *Prometheus*, 27, 47–70.

Winch, P. (1963). *The Idea of a Social Science and Its Relation to Philosophy.* (First published 1958). London: Routledge & Kegan Paul.

Wittchen, H.U. & Jacobi, F. (2005). Size and burden of mental disorders in Europe: A critical review and appraisal of 27 studies. *European Neuropsychopharmacology,* 15, 357–376.

Wittchen, H.U., Jacobi, F., & Rehm, J., et al. (2011). The size and burden of mental disorders and other disorders of the brain in Europe 2012. *European Neuropsychopharmacology,* 21, 655–679.

Wittgenstein, L. (1953). *Philosophical Investigations.* Oxford: Basil Blackwell.

Wykes, T. & Callard, F. (2010). Diagnosis, diagnosis, diagnosis: Towards DSM-5. *Journal of Mental Health,* 19, 301–304.

Young, S., Bramham, J., Gray, K., & Rose, E. (2008). The experience of receiving a diagnosis and treatment of ADHD in adulthood. *Journal of Attention Disorders,* 11, 493–503.

Zittoun, T. (2006). *Transitions: Development through Symbolic Resources.* Greenwich: Information Age Publishing.

Index

Bold page numbers indicate figures.

Printed in the United States
by Baker & Taylor Publisher Services